WHAT YOUR DOCTOR DOESN'T KNOW ABOUT
NUTRITIONAL MEDICINE MAY BE KILLING YOU

WHAT YOUR DOCTOR DOESN'T KNOW ABOUT NUTRITIONAL MEDICINE MAY BE KILLING YOU

Ray D. Strand, M.D.

with Donna K. Wallace

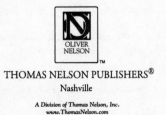

THOMAS NELSON PUBLISHERS®
Nashville

A Division of Thomas Nelson, Inc.
www.ThomasNelson.com

Published in Nashville, Tennessee, by Thomas Nelson, Inc.

Scripture quotations are from the NEW AMERICAN STANDARD BIBLE®, © Copyright The Lockman Foundation 1960, 1962, 1963, 1968, 1971, 1972, 1973, 1975, 1977. Used by permission.

Library of Congress Cataloging-in-Publication Data

Strand, Ray D.
    What your doctor doesn't know about nutritional medicine may be killing you / by Ray D. Strand.
      p. cm.
    ISBN: 0-7852-6486-8
    1. Dietary supplements—Popular works. 2. Diet in disease—Popular works. 3. Alternative medicine—Popular works.
    [DNLM: 1. Dietary Supplements—Popular Works. 2. Complementary Therapies—Popular Works. 3. Diet Therapy—Popular Works. QU 145.5 S897w 2002] I. Title.
RM258.5 .S77 2002   2002007202

Printed in the United States of America

02 03 04 05 06 BVG 5 4 3

This book is written with deep humility and respect for the Great Physician.

• • •

It is with great awe and appreciation that I dedicate this book to the most beautiful display of God's handiwork: my wife, Elizabeth.

Contents

Beloved, I pray that in all respects you may prosper and be in good health, just as your soul prospers.

—3 JOHN 2

Acknowledgments

First, there are no words to adequately acknowledge the wonderful grace that my Redeemer has given me. He is the Great Physician, and He is the one who truly heals. Each day I am astounded by the knowledge of His handiwork as I learn more about the body's great ability to protect and heal itself.

There are many individuals who have come together to make this book a reality and whom I greatly appreciate. I express my deepest thanks to my agent, Kathryn Helmers, who has guided me faithfully through this entire project; to my publishers, Victor Oliver and Michael Hyatt at Thomas Nelson, who recognized the potentially life-changing health concepts presented in this book; to Kristen Lucas, my managing editor, whose attention to the details of this project made it all happen; to Alice Crider, for her careful creation of the index.

I want to give a special thanks to my collaborator, Donna Wallace, whose wonderful talent and influence is seen throughout this book. Without her energy and guidance, this project would never have seen completion.

My entire clinic staff has been wonderful. I need especially to thank my two nurse practitioners, Paulette Nankivel and Melissa Aberle, for graciously allowing me the extra time necessary to write this book. I must also thank Karmen Thompson and Leone Young, who helped me gather the volumes of medical research that provide the facts and foundation of this work.

I want especially to thank Bruce Nygren, whose support actually gave me the opportunity to write this book. My prayers go out to Bruce, who lost his lovely wife, Racinda, during the writing of this book.

Words cannot express the love and support I have received from my wife, Elizabeth, whose encouragement has buoyed me up during the long hours of research and writing. And to my children, Donny, Nick, and Sarah, who are all grown but offer continual support and encouragement: thank you.

Introduction

PHYSICIANS ARE DISEASE-ORIENTED. WE STUDY DISEASE. WE LOOK for disease. We are pharmaceutically trained to treat disease. And in order to do so, we know our drugs. In medical school we study pharmacology and learn how the body absorbs each drug, and when and how the body excretes it. We know which drugs disrupt certain chemical pathways to create a therapeutic effect. We learn the side-effect profiles of drugs, and we work carefully to balance the benefits against any potential danger.

Physicians know their drugs and don't hesitate to prescribe them. Consider for a moment the number of drugs that our patients are taking for high blood pressure, elevated cholesterol, diabetes mellitus, arthritis, heart disease, and depression, to name just a few. As a result of the discovery and use of antibiotics in the war against infectious disease, our philosophy in medicine has become: *attack disease.*

The medical community has carried this aggressive attitude and approach into the twenty-first century in the attempt to treat all the various chronic degenerative diseases. A study estimates that in 1997, pharmacies filled more than 2.5 billion retail prescriptions in the United States alone. The sale of prescription drugs has more than doubled in just the past eight years![1]

In 1990 Americans spent $37.7 billion on prescriptions. In 1997 that spending increased to $78.9 billion. Prescription drugs have been the fastest-growing portion of health-care costs over the past decade, rising at the rate of about 17 percent per year (well above the average rate of inflation).[2] Physicians and insurance companies have placed all their hopes in drugs as the way to approach and hopefully slow down this epidemic of chronic degenerative disease—much to the delight of the pharmaceutical industry. Yes—we love our drugs.

I have not met a person yet who does not want to have excellent health. Most of us assume that we always will. But the truth is that many of us (doctors included!) are losing our health each day. I know, because health care is my job. Every day of my career involves informing patients that they have lost their health in one aspect or another. One patient may have developed diabetes or maybe degenerative arthritis. Another patient may have just suffered a heart attack or stroke. Still another may have to be told that he has metastatic cancer and has only a few months to live. Everyone desires to maintain or regain his health, but he does not always know what he needs to do to achieve that goal.

Because physicians are disease- and drug-oriented, we spend most of our time and effort trying to identify a disease process so we can prescribe a drug or treatment plan for our patient. Even Jesus made the statement, "It is not those who are healthy who need a physician, but those who are sick."[3]

Yet it just makes common sense that it is much easier to maintain our health than to try to regain it after it has been lost. Prevention of disease should be the first order of business for any physician. But to whom do you actually turn when you want to learn about the best way to *protect* your health? Is your doctor providing you with this information? The medical community gives plenty of lip service to "preventive medicine" and even names its leading medical insurance plans HMOs (Health Maintenance Organizations). By all appearances preventive medicine seems to be a top priority.

Yet less than 1 percent of our health-care dollars are spent on so-called preventive medicine. In reality the majority of our preventive medicine programs simply attempt to detect disease earlier. For example, mammograms, chemistry profiles, and PSA tests (for prostate cancer) are all designed to detect a problem or cancer as early as possible. Doctors want to know if you have elevated cholesterol, whether you have become diabetic or developed hypertension. But they spend very little time trying to help the patient understand the lifestyle changes that are necessary to actually protect his or her health. Physicians are too busy treating all the disease they face each day.

Are you aware that less than 6 percent of graduating physicians receive any formal training in nutrition?[4] And I would boldly state that few physicians receive training in medical school in regard to nutritional supplementation. This was certainly true in my case.

Nothing curls a physician's toes more readily than the moment his patient asks if he should be taking nutritional supplements. I've used all the patented answers in the past: "They're just snake oil." "Vitamins just make expensive urine." "You can get all the required nutrients by eating the right foods." If my patients persisted, I told them nutritional supplements probably would not hurt them, but they should take the cheapest ones they could find because vitamins most likely wouldn't help much either.

Maybe you have heard some of these same comments from your physician. For the first twenty-three years of my clinical practice, I simply did not believe in nutritional supplements. During the past seven years, however, I have reconsidered my position based on recent studies published in the medical literature. What I've found is so astonishing, I have changed the course of my medical practice. I have converted.

Why aren't more doctors responding to nutrition as I have? First, physicians must be skeptical in order to protect their patients against any scheme or product that could be harmful to their health. Believe me, I have seen plenty of gimmicks and quackery peddled to my patients. Physicians must rely on scientific research studies conducted through double-blind, placebo-controlled clinical trials (the standard in clinical medicine).

Because I know it's the most effective evidence available, I present only clinical trial study results in this book. Most of the medical studies I offer here are not from abstract or alternative journals. Instead, I have painstakingly researched mainstream, credible medical journals that the medical community greatly respects, such as the *New England Journal of Medicine, Journal of the American Medical Association, British Lancet*, and many others.

Another reason doctors haven't accepted the nutritional supplement idea as good preventive medicine is that most practicing physicians don't fully understand the cause of degenerative diseases. Those who do often feel this is an interesting subject for the biochemist and scientific researchers, but it has little in the way of practical use in clinical medicine. An apparent chasm exists between the research scientist and the practicing physician. Even though research scientists are making tremendous discoveries into the root causes of these diseases, very few physicians are applying this science to their patients. Doctors simply wait until patients develop one of these diseases and then begin to treat it.

Physicians seem content to allow the pharmaceutical companies to determine new therapies as they develop new drugs. But as you will learn throughout this book, it is our own bodies that are the best defense against developing a chronic degenerative disease—not the drugs doctors can prescribe.

Though most physicians do not yet well understand the concepts presented here, the facts remain. As I have applied these principles in treating my patients, the results have been nothing short of amazing. I have been involved with numerous patients with multiple sclerosis who have gone from being wheelchair-bound to walking again. I have helped patients with cardiomyopathy get off the heart-transplant list. Some cancer patients have gone into remission; patients with macular degeneration have had significant visual improvement; and fibromyalgia patients have gotten their lives back. Nutritional medicine is common-sense, mainstream, preventive medicine.

In this age of biochemical research, we are now able to determine what is happening in every part of each cell, and the very essence of degenerative diseases is now coming to light. As such, I recommend this book to physicians who are willing to look objectively at medical evidence.

If you are a patient, don't expect your physician to jump onto the bandwagon immediately. Vitamins are a hot issue within the medical field. *What Your Doctor Doesn't Know* is, as I said, the outcome of more than *seven years* of personal research into the medical literature as it pertains to nutritional medicine. I wasn't immediately convinced either.

Nutritional medicine is foreign to most physicians as well as the public; this is true. But the verdict is in: *what your doctor doesn't know about nutritional medicine may be killing you.* The good news is that you do not have to be a physician to start practicing nutritional medicine; you, the patient, can become proactive about preserving the health you have.

A Converted Doctor

I know that you probably have never heard of me. Why should you take the word of some doctor who practices medicine in a small city in the Midwest? Good question! That's why I want you to read every page in this book. I want you to undertake a journey similar to mine. Let me show you the same medical evidence that made me believe that vitamin supplements can protect and improve health.

Please do read or at least scan the *entire book*. I know the temptation is to jump ahead to the specific chapter that discusses your health problem. But it is important that you become aware of the foundational information on how your body functions and what it needs to protect itself and become or stay healthy.

One final request: Since it's your health and life that are at stake, I encourage you to hear me out and withhold judgment. All I ask is that you be an open-minded skeptic—the kind of seeker I was when I first discovered this wondrous form of preventive medicine. I had to humble myself a bit to learn that even though I was a good doctor I had much to learn about health. Are you willing to do the same?

PART I

BEFORE YOU BEGIN

ONE | My Conversion

I WAS NOT SURE HOW MUCH MORE FRUSTRATION I COULD BEAR OVER my wife's deteriorating health. And I wasn't just another worried husband; I was a medical doctor. As a physician for more than thirty years, I was accustomed to having answers to medical questions. After graduating from the University of Colorado Medical School and doing postgraduate work at Mercy Hospital in San Diego, I settled into a successful family practice in a small city in western South Dakota. Along the way I met and married Liz. She had some health problems, but Liz honestly thought that if she married a physician her health would improve. Was she ever wrong!

Before long our family included three children under the age of four and a busy Liz grew increasingly weary. Every mom with little children is tired, but Liz seemed unusually fatigued. Although she was only thirty years old, she told me she felt sixty.

As the years passed she developed more symptoms and health problems that required several medications. By our tenth anniversary Liz was so tired that most of the time she labored to put one foot ahead of the other. She experienced continual, total body pain, overwhelming fatigue, horrible allergies, and recurrent sinus and lung infections.

Finally, after testing and evaluation, Liz's doctors diagnosed her problem as fibromyalgia. This medical condition involves an array of symptoms—the worst being chronic pain and fatigue.

In years past fibromyalgia was called *psychosomatic rheumatism*, and doctors believed the disease was all in the patient's head. We have since learned that fibromyalgia is a true, miserable disease—which I can vouch for after watching my wife suffer.

Liz was willing to try anything so that she could continue the pursuit of her passion: training and riding dressage horses. But in time her pain and fatigue curtailed all work with her beloved animals. She became so severely tired that she was unable to stay up much beyond 8:00 P.M., and she struggled just to keep up with basic domestic chores.

Since fibromyalgia has no cure, all I could do to ease Liz's symptoms was load her up with medications. I had her taking amitriptyline at night for sleep, anti-inflammatories for pain, muscle relaxants, inhalers for her asthma and hay fever, seldane for allergies, and eventually weekly allergy shots. In spite of my efforts and all this medicine, year after year her health gradually worsened.

In January of 1995 Liz and I concluded that more exercise would benefit us both. We had put on extra pounds and made a New Year's resolution to get back into shape. Liz tried hard but missed more workouts than she made. One infection after another left her sick and on antibiotics more often than not.

In March she developed a severe pneumonia. She labored to breathe as one lobe of her lungs became completely filled with infection and closed off. The physician caring for her lung was very concerned it might not heal and could possibly even require surgery and removal. We consulted an infectious-disease specialist, and he placed Liz on intravenous antibiotics, steroids, and nebulizer treatments. Fortunately, within two weeks the pneumonia cleared. Her cough, however, persisted, and she continued on heavy medication for months.

Of greater concern was her fatigue, which was now worse than ever. Liz was out of bed only about two hours a day. Her asthma and allergies were raging and only with luck could she make the walk to the barn to see her horses. Liz was so sick the children took turns staying home from school to care for her. Constantly in bed, she felt too weak even to watch TV or read. This went on month after month. Although I maintained my professional exterior, on the inside I was growing desperate.

I visited several times with the pulmonologist and the infectious-disease specialist. They assured me that with Liz's diagnosis they were doing everything possible. When I asked how long it would take for her to recover, the answer was six to nine months—or maybe never.

About this time a friend of the family shared with Liz that her husband had also had pneumonia and had experienced significant fatigue during the recovery. He took some nutritional supplements, and they had helped him regain his strength. Liz and her friend were aware of my negative attitude toward vitamin supplements, so Liz knew she would need my blessing before trying them. When she asked, even I was surprised at my response: "Honey, you can try anything you want. We doctors certainly are not doing you any good."

Presuppositions Put to the Test

To be honest, I knew next to nothing about nutrition or nutritional supplementation. In medical school I had not received any significant instruction on the subject. I was not alone. Only approximately 6 percent of the graduating physicians in the United States have any training in nutrition. Medical students may take elective courses on the topic, but few actually do. As I mentioned in the introduction, the education of most physicians is disease-oriented with a heavy emphasis on pharmaceuticals—we learn about drugs and why and when to use them.

Because of the respect people have for doctors, they assume we are experts on all health-related issues, including nutrition and vitamins. Before my conversion experience with nutritional medicine, my patients frequently asked me if I believed their taking vitamins produced any health benefits. They brought their bottles of supplements into the office and let me look at them. I'd wrinkle my brow and, with my most astute professional expression, would carefully examine the labels. Handing the bottles back, I'd say that the stuff was absolutely no use at all.

My motives were good: I just didn't want people wasting their money. I truly believed that these patients did not need supplements and could get all the vitamins they needed from a good diet. After all, that's what I had learned in medical school. I could even quote a few research studies that showed the potential danger of some supplements. What I did not share with my patients was that I had not spent a minute evaluating the hundreds of scientifically conducted studies that proved the value of supplementation to health.

But what was I to do about my sickly wife? I might be able to pull off professional magic at the office, but at home I was just another husband looking on helplessly as his wife wasted away. I really had no choice, so I said to Liz, "Go ahead, try the vitamins. What do you have to lose?"

Her friend brought a collection of vitamin supplements to our house the next day—heavy on the antioxidants: nutrients like vitamin E, vitamin C, and beta-carotene that protect the body against the harmful effects of oxidation. Liz eagerly swallowed them and downed two health drinks as well. To my amazement, within three days she obviously felt better. I was happy for her but confused. As subsequent days passed, Liz gained more energy and strength and even stayed up later in the evenings. After three weeks of faithfully swallowing many pills and consuming those strange-looking drinks, Liz felt so good that she stopped taking the steroids and nebulizer treatments.

Three months passed, all bringing gradual improvement, and Liz never looked back. She was stronger than she had been in years and exuded a renewed outlook on life. I saw the sparkle in her eyes when she returned from training and caring for her horses. She not only could do the work in the horse barn but also was no longer fearful of suffering from allergic reactions to the hay, mold, and dust. Instead of limping off to bed shortly after dinner, she was staying up until 11:00 and 12:00 at night. I was now the one who headed to bed before my mate.

What had happened? I was dumbfounded. If I had not been an eyewitness to this transformation, I would have never believed it. Was it possible that some "weird vitamins" had restored my wife's health when all the medical expertise and medications could not help? Not only had Liz's lungs recovered from the pneumonia, the symptoms of her fibromyalgia had improved dramatically. Since there really is no medical treatment for fibromyalgia, what was going on? Was this one of God's mysterious miracles or was it possible that Liz's newly recovered health was due to those—*horror*—nutritional supplements?

For a person trained in medical science I did what comes naturally: I decided to run my own clinical trial. I culled my records to find five of my worst fibromyalgia patients and asked them to visit my office. (How's that for a twist—a doctor calling a patient to make an appointment?) I shared Liz's story with all of them and suggested they consider taking nutritional supplements. I told each patient that I had no idea whether this "alternative treatment" would help, but it was worth a try.

Typical fibromyalgia sufferers are despondent, so each of my five subjects was very eager. After a period of time ranging from three to six months, without exception each patient reported improvement after taking the vitamin supplements. Not everyone had as dramatic a health rebound as my wife, but all were encouraged and had fresh hope.

One of these women's cases was particularly severe. She had sought answers at the Mayo Clinic and two different pain clinics, but because there really is no effective medical treatment for fibromyalgia, she found no consistent relief. A year earlier pain had so beaten her down that she had attempted suicide. Now, after taking these vitamins, she called and left a message on my home answering machine. Obviously in tears and struggling to speak, she said: "Dr. Strand, thank you for giving my life back to me."

Every doctor loves to hear words like that. But just what was happening to these patients? Since I knew that my preliminary study with five patients was not enough to reach scientific certainty on nutritional supplements, I needed to dig deeper.

My Research on Supplementation

While browsing through a bookstore a week later, I saw a book by Dr. Kenneth Cooper called *The Antioxidant Revolution* (Thomas Nelson, 1994). Since I had always admired Dr. Cooper for his expertise on aerobic exercise and preventative medicine, I was inquisitive about his opinions on antioxidants. Dr. Cooper explained a process called "oxidative stress," which he indicated was the underlying cause of chronic degenerative diseases—essentially a "who's who" of the health problems plaguing humanity today. I devoured the book.

We all know that oxygen is essential for life itself. Yet oxygen is also inherently dangerous to our existence. This is known as the *oxygen paradox*. Scientific research has established beyond a shadow of doubt that oxidative stress, or cell damage by free radicals, is the root cause of more than seventy chronic degenerative diseases.[2] The same process that causes iron to rust or a cut apple to turn brown is the underlying initiator of diseases like coronary artery disease, cancer, strokes, arthritis, multiple sclerosis, Alzheimer's dementia, and macular degeneration.

That is right: we are actually rusting on the inside. Every chronic degenerative disease I have mentioned is the direct result of the toxic effects of oxygen. In fact oxidative stress is the leading theory behind the aging process itself. In addition to this, our bodies are under constant attack from an army of pollutants in our air, food, and water. Our stress-filled lifestyles also take a toll. If we do not counteract these processes, the result is cell deterioration and ultimately, disease. This is why the truths revealed in this book are so critical to our health.

Learning about how unhindered oxidative stress damages the body drastically changed my perspective on chronic degenerative diseases. For example, since oxidative stress can actually cause damage to the DNA nucleus of the cell, it may be the actual villain in cancer. This opens up the tremendous possibility of using antioxidants in cancer prevention. Since oxidative stress also causes arthritis, multiple sclerosis, lupus, macular degeneration, diabetes, Parkinson's disease, and Crohn's disease, nutritional supplements may also combat and control those illnesses.

In his book Dr. Cooper reported on some studies of patients done at his aerobics center in Dallas concerning the cause of "overtraining syndrome." Surprisingly, Dr. Cooper discovered that some athletes who trained intensely ended up later struggling with serious chronic illness. They all showed signs of having oxidative stress, and the list of the symptoms associated with the syndrome were eerily similar to those of fibromyalgia patients.[3]

I began to wonder, *Could oxidative stress cause fibromyalgia too? Is this why my wife and several of my patients are getting better by taking high-quality antioxidants?*

This marked the beginning of my investigation into the "dark side" of oxygen. I was so intrigued by Dr. Cooper's arguments that I decided to check out the research studies he had cited. I started a search for everything I could find in mainstream medical literature on oxidative stress.

In the past year alone, I have examined more than thirteen hundred peer-reviewed medical studies involving nutritional supplements and how they affect chronic degenerative diseases. These studies are double-blind, placebo-controlled medical studies, the kind that physicians love. The overwhelming majority of these studies show a significant health benefit to those patients who take nutrients at optimal levels, which are significantly higher than the RDA (recommended daily allowance) levels.

Vitamins and You

When you understand the tremendous damage that oxidative stress inflicts during normal daily life on the human body, you realize how important it is to optimize your own natural defense system. Your health and life depend on it. Through my research I learned that the strongest defense against these diseases is our bodies' own natural antioxidant and immune systems. These are far superior to any drugs I can prescribe.

I concluded after much study that using nutritional supplementation on patients is not alternative medicine but is instead complementary medicine.

In fact it may represent the very best in mainline medicine because it is true preventive medicine. Taking nutritional supplements is not about eradicating disease; it is about promoting vibrant health.

After reviewing medical research studies, I have absolutely no doubt that my patients who take high-quality nutritional supplements have a health benefit over those who don't. Although a patient may have a particular health problem, in recommending supplements I am not necessarily treating that particular disease. I am simply enabling the patient to provide the nutrients to his or her body at the optimal levels that studies have shown to provide a health benefit based on medical research. This approach to health I have labeled *cellular nutrition,* which enables the body to do what God intended.

The personal case histories that I present in this book are ones I have documented in my office. I've changed some names to protect privacy, but many are the stories of patients and friends who wanted to share the exact details of their stories here with you. Within these stories you will discover real-life examples of how the important concepts I present were actually applied.

If you are already sick, please be encouraged. Almost all of these true stories are about patients who had lost their health too. With much courage and determination they continued to seek answers, and after testing the principles presented here, they regained their health.

Liz is my best case study. By the way, her health remains robust—even though she married a doctor! Instead of spending many hours of every day in pain and weakness in bed, she now lives the full life of her dreams. She has the energy to fully enjoy being a wife and mother. And her passion for training and showing horses is no longer just wishful thinking but a daily reality.

To learn more about this amazing form of preventive medicine, read on.

TWO | Living Too Short; Dying Too Long

AS WE ROUNDED THE CORNER INTO THE TWENTY-FIRST CENTURY, physicians and medical researchers took special note of the state of health and medical care in the United States and the industrialized world. Looking back over a century gone by, the comparisons of diseases are remarkable. In the early 1900s people primarily died of *infectious* diseases. The four leading of causes of death in the U.S. back then were pneumonia, tuberculosis, diphtheria, and influenza, and people had a life expectancy of a little more than forty-three years. But thanks to the discovery of antibiotics and advances in their development during the second half of this century, deaths due to infectious diseases declined dramatically, even after the AIDS epidemic of the 1980s.[1]

As we move into the twenty-first century, we find people primarily suffering and dying from what are known as *chronic degenerative diseases*. These include coronary artery disease, cancer, stroke, diabetes, arthritis, macular degeneration, cataracts, Alzheimer's dementia, Parkinson's disease, multiple sclerosis, and rheumatoid arthritis.[2] The list goes on and on.

Even though the average life expectancy in the United States has increased dramatically during this past century, our quality of life due to these chronic degenerative diseases has taken a major hit. We are essentially "living too short and dying too long," as I heard expressed in a speech by Dr. Myron Wentz, a prominent immunologist and microbiologist. Dr. Wentz also helped me understand the serious danger of oxidative stress to our health and the importance of cellular nutrition.

A Wake-Up Call

Life Expectancy

How long do you expect to live? Let's set aside the quality of life for a moment (as do many research studies on longevity) and consider how the U.S. compares with all the other industrialized nations in the world when it comes to life expectancy and health care. One of the primary ways to evaluate a nation's health-care system is to look at the death rate of that country.

In 1950 the United States ranked *seventh* among the top twenty-one industrialized nations in the world when it came to life expectancy. As you might imagine, we have spent far more money on health care since that time than any other country in the world. In 1998 we spent more than $1 trillion on health care, averaging 13.6 percent of our gross national product. That is more than twice as much as the next closest nation.[3] We have our MRI and CT scanners, angioplasty, bypass surgery, total hip and knee replacement, chemotherapy, radiation therapy, antibiotics, advanced surgical techniques, advanced drugs, and intensive care units. Did all our medical advances increase U.S. life expectancy?

In 1990 our nation ranked *eighteenth* in life expectancy when compared to the same twenty-one industrialized nations forty years prior.[4] In spite of the billions of dollars Americans spend on health care, we are now considered one of the worst industrialized nations in the world when it comes to life expectancy. The health-care system we claim is the best in the world is actually near the worst when we look at how long Americans live—or don't live.

I asked how long you expect to live, but now envision what your last twenty years will look like. Are you getting your money's worth? I don't think so.

Quality of Life

I can assure you that my patients today are not as concerned with the number of years in their lives as they are with the quality of life in those years. Are you? The number of years we live is not usually the most important consideration when it comes to evaluating our approach to health care. Who wants to live to a ripe old age if he cannot even recognize his closest family member because he has Alzheimer's dementia? Who looks forward to suffering severe joint or back pain because of degenerative arthritis? Our nation is suffering from Parkinson's disease, macular degeneration, cancer, strokes, and heart disease with unprecedented frequency. No one seems to die of *old age* anymore.

More than 60 million Americans suffer from some form of cardiovascular disease (disease of the heart and blood vessels); more than 13.6 million have coronary artery disease. Although a decrease has occurred in the number of cardiovascular deaths in the past twenty-five years, it still remains the number-one cause of death in the United States. There are 1.5 million heart attacks each year and about one-half, or just over seven hundred thousand, are fatal. Sadly, about half of these deaths occur within the first hour of a heart attack and long before the individual can even make it to the hospital. The first sign of heart disease in more than 30 percent of cases is sudden death.[5] This does not give us much time to make lifestyle changes.

In spite of the tremendous amount of money spent on cancer research and treatment, cancer remains the second leading cause of death in the United States. There were 537,000 cancer deaths in 1995; there has been a steady increase in the number of deaths caused by cancer over the past thirty years.[6]

The U.S. has spent more than $25 billion in cancer research over the past twenty-five years only to see absolutely no decrease in the relative number of people dying from cancer. The greatest advancements in cancer treatment have developed because of earlier diagnoses of certain cancers—not that our treatments for cancer have been pleasant or overly effective.[7]

My patients with macular degeneration, a chronic disease affecting eyesight, visit their ophthalmologist every six months only to have to make another appointment six months down the road. They become frustrated knowing that the only thing their doctor is able to do is document the progression of their disease. In some cases laser treatment may have only minimal effect.

If you have a loved one who is suffering from Alzheimer's dementia, you are acutely aware of the ineffectiveness of treatments. Watching a parent slowly lose any reasonable function of mind and become trapped in his or her own body is extremely painful.

It's time to go back to the drawing board. If we physicians are truly honest with ourselves, we have to admit that the treatment options we offer many of these patients are poor at best. We are not able to attack these ailments the way we did with infectious diseases. Doctors and patients alike must take a long, hard look at how they approach health care today.

Preventive Medicine

I find disturbing the overwhelming attitude in patients today that accepts as inevitable the fact that they are going to develop one or several of these chronic degenerative diseases. They look to modern medicine as their savior and to medications as the cure. Sadly, only after they become ill do patients realize how ineffective our treatments actually are.

As the baby boomer generation enters their fifties, I believe more and more individuals are going to become proactive with their health.

One of my close friends told me last month that he simply wants to live until he dies. Is this your desire? It certainly is mine. After practicing medicine for more than three decades, I find greatly disturbing the prospects of the pain and suffering that chronic degenerative diseases can bring to both myself and my patients.

That's why I wrote this book; that's why I recommend preventive rather than post-problem medicine. But I need to define what I mean by *preventive*.

Traditional Preventive Medicine (Early Detection)

The health-care community prides itself on promoting preventive care. But have you ever given that approach much thought? Physicians certainly do encourage patients to have routine physicals in order to maintain their health. But a closer look into doctors' helpful recommendations quickly leads one to the conclusion that they are simply attempting to detect disease *earlier*. Think about it. As I've mentioned physicians routinely perform pap smears, mammograms, blood work, and the physical exam primarily to see if any silent diseases already exist in their patients. *What has been prevented?*

Obviously the earlier these diseases are detected, the better it is for the patient. The point I want to stress here, however, is the minimal time and effort the physician or the health-care community actually gives to teaching patients how they can *protect* their health. In other words physicians are simply too busy treating disease to worry about educating their patients in healthy lifestyles that help avoid developing degenerative diseases in the first place.

True Preventive Medicine

If we are going to label something *preventive*, then I believe it should actually prevent something. I strongly suggest that true preventive medicine involves encouraging and supporting patients to take a threefold approach: eating healthily, practicing a consistent exercise program, and consuming high-quality nutritional supplements. Empowering patients to avoid getting some of these major diseases in the first place is true prevention.

Does it require patient motivation? Absolutely. But most people are very willing to make these lifestyle changes when they truly understand what is at stake.

This is where I feel the medical field has fallen short: in practicing true preventive medicine.

The Ingredients of a Healthy Lifestyle

Exercise

We have forgotten about the "host," our bodies, being one of our greatest defenses against becoming ill. I find Dr. Kenneth Cooper to be one of the leading physicians in the field of preventive medicine. He coined the term *aerobics* and began the exercise craze in the early 1970s.

Today we all take as gospel truth a fact that had to be medically proven just three decades ago. I remember physicians arguing in meetings back then about whether encouraging their patients to exercise was the right thing to do. Dr. Cooper was insistent and continued to share the health benefits that exercising could bring to the patient. By the end of the seventies, most physicians agreed with Dr. Cooper and began recommending a modest exercise program.

The surgeon general of the United States issued a statement in the early 1980s listing all the major health benefits that result from a modest exercise program. The highlights of these benefits are:

- weight loss.
- lower blood pressure.
- stronger bones and a decreased risk of osteoporosis.
- elevated levels of "good" HDL cholesterol.
- decreased levels of "bad" LDL cholesterol.
- decreased levels of triglycerides (fats).
- increased strength and coordination, which leads to a decrease in the risk of falls.
- improved sensitivity to insulin.
- enhancement of the immune system.
- overall increase in one's sense of well-being.

One look at this list of health benefits is convincing: any individual who chooses to develop a consistent program of modest exercise is making an important choice to avoid developing many different diseases.

Healthy Diet

What about eating habits? Physicians also realize that patients who eat a low-fat diet, which includes at least seven servings of fruits and vegetables daily, enjoy further health benefits. These include:

- weight loss.
- a decreased risk of diabetes.
- a decreased risk of heart disease.
- a decreased risk of almost all cancers.
- a decreased risk of high blood pressure.
- a decreased risk of elevated cholesterol.
- an enhanced immune system.
- an increased sensitivity to insulin.
- increased energy and ability to concentrate.

Let's face it: a healthy diet is a win/win situation!

Nutritional Supplements

As I have researched the medical literature over the past seven years, I strongly believe that there are significant health benefits in taking high-quality nutritional supplements, even if you are in excellent health. Put simply, the basic health benefits of nutritional supplements are:

- an enhanced immune system.
- an enhanced antioxidant defense system.
- a decreased risk of coronary artery disease.
- a decreased risk of stroke.
- a decreased risk of cancer.

- a decreased risk of arthritis, macular degeneration, and cataracts.

- the potential for a decreased risk of Alzheimer's dementia, Parkinson's disease, asthma, obstructive lung disease, and many other chronic degenerative diseases.

- the potential for improving the clinical course of several chronic degenerative diseases.

Could patients who begin a consistent exercise program and a healthy diet while taking supplements actually improve their high blood pressure, diabetes, and high cholesterol to the point of being able to avoid taking some medications? The medical literature certainly supports this approach.

Almost all physicians agree that patients deserve a fair trial of healthy lifestyle changes before beginning medication for such chronic conditions. In reality, however, most physicians merely give lip service to lifestyle changes in their office even as they are writing out prescriptions. You see, doctors usually assume that most patients will never change their lifestyles and the only realistic salvation is the drugs they can prescribe. When a physician first diagnoses a patient with high blood pressure, diabetes, or elevated cholesterol, he simply begins writing a prescription.

Giving Patients a Choice

Over the past seven or eight years, I have taken a different attitude: I use medication as a last resort—not as my first choice. I have been amazed at how many of my patients are actually willing to become more proactive with their health if even a slight chance exists that they could avoid taking any medication. Oh, sure, I still have those patients who do not consider changing. For them, I still have the drugs.

There are also those patients whose condition is serious enough that I have to start them on medication right away. But I also offer those individuals a chance to improve their condition over time with healthy lifestyle changes in the hopes that they may someday be able to decrease or discontinue their medication.

Everyone knows about the health benefits of a good exercise program and a healthy diet. Few, however (especially physicians), have any knowledge of the health benefits of taking high-quality nutritional supplements. I've mentioned that I was one of those uninformed doctors. But countless studies prove that this triad of a healthy diet, a good exercise program, and high-quality nutritional supplements is the absolute best way you can protect your health. It is also the best way to try to regain your health after you have lost it.

David's Story

Let's see the theory at work. "David" had spent most of his life as a driver's license examiner in the state of Utah, where he lived with his wife and children. David had always enjoyed excellent health and wasn't on any medication. Early in 1990, however, he began noting weakness in his legs associated with unusual fatigue. By the spring of 1990, he was dragging his legs and actually falling from time to time. He had been seeing several different doctors, and a neurologist finally diagnosed him as having a rare disease called *leukoencephalopathy.*

I am sure David responded to the name of his disease much the way you are: *What is that?* The neurologist informed him that it was a progressive, degenerative, demyelinating disease of the brain, quite similar to multiple sclerosis, for which no real treatment is available. The physician told David there was very little hope for him—this disease usually pursued a relentless downhill course to death.

The news devastated David. He returned home despondent and shocked. He had never heard of this disease, and now it was going to take his life. True to the doctor's words, David became weaker. He started developing vertigo and began to lose control of his bowels and bladder. By the spring of 1993, David was wheelchair-bound. By June of 1995 the pain in his legs was so extreme that his doctors put him on an oral form of morphine. He was now totally dependent on his wife and kids for everything. Life as he had known it was gone.

In November of 1995 David came down with a serious case of influenza. David became even weaker and his legs and arms grew cold, as if they had no circulation. His doctors informed David and his family that he would not likely recover. Because of the underlying leukoencephalopathy, they expected him to live only a week or two.

David had been under the care of the Hospice Program, which allowed him to stay home where he wanted to be. He and his family began making funeral plans. David grieved the loss of all that he loved while saying good-bye to family and friends. Though he had accepted his death a couple years before, the time had finally come, just as the doctors predicted.

But somehow David lived through Christmas. Although he was not able to get out of bed, he didn't die either.

A couple of months later David decided to try some nutritional supplements. He started on an antioxidant tablet, a mineral tablet, and some grape-seed extract. Within five days he was sleeping less and noted that he had a little more energy. After several weeks of taking the supplements he was able to get out of bed for short intervals. In fact on Mother's Day his children pushed him down to the flower shop so he could do his traditional shopping for his wife and mother. Week after week, David regained hope as he grew stronger and stronger.

David remembers watching the movie *Lorenzo's Oil* in the summer of 1996. The little boy in the movie, Lorenzo, had a brain disease similar to David's. While watching the movie, David was astounded to discover that the most important part of Lorenzo's treatment, the one that actually seemed to hinder his decline, was grape-seed oil. David realized that his own use of grape-seed extract could be a major factor in his marked improvement. He decided at that moment to start taking more of it. He soon learned that the extract is a very potent antioxidant, which the fluid around the brain can easily absorb. David's improvement after increasing the amount of grape-seed extract, while continuing with the other antioxidants and minerals, was amazing. The pain in his legs began to subside, and he actually began to walk again. The strength in his legs increased consistently week after week. About two months later, David was able to walk into church on his own for the first time in three years. He still had a significant shuffle to his walk, but he was walking!

David's physician stopped the morphine prescription and documented his patient's improvement. While he couldn't believe it, the doctor couldn't deny it either. David's greatest thrill was when he was able to go back and take his driver's license exam and actually pass. After all those years of testing others, he was able to drive by himself again.

David still has his disease. He is not cured. But he, rather than the disease, is in control of his life. He still has a funny walk, but he doesn't mind. Every time I see David I have to smile. It has been a delight watching his progress.

He is one the many reasons I am positive the use of nutritional medicine holds so much promise for patients in all types of health.

•   •   •

In this chapter we've discussed our nation's approach to health care. What is yours? Do you fear growing old? Have you accepted chronic disease or pain as a given in your future? Are you willing to make necessary life changes to ensure your health? I believe a full and abundant physical life does not need to start slipping away at age forty. I believe each year of your life can be your very best. It is time to stop living too short and dying too long! But first you must understand the war that is waging within every one of our bodies.

We'll cover that next.

THREE | The War Within

Sit back, close your eyes for a moment, and focus on your breathing. Relax your shoulders and breathe in as deeply as you can, and then slowly release the air from your lungs. Do this several times. Breathe as if you are inflating your whole body, clear down to your toes. Pause and then slowly exhale. Feels great, doesn't it? The air that enters our lungs brings life. And as we quicken our breathing through aerobic exercise or running, we feel invigorated and may even experience a feeling of euphoria.

Being a doctor, I like to imagine what is happening inside my body at a cellular level as oxygen enters through my nose and travels to my lungs. Life is an intricately woven miracle, evident in every breath. I fill my lungs with fresh air rich with oxygen. The molecules of oxygen then pass through the thin walls of the alveoli in the lungs into the blood that is passing by. Here it attaches itself to the hemoglobin in my blood, and my beating heart pumps this newly oxygenated blood back out to all parts of my body. The hemoglobin then releases the oxygen so it can enter the cells of my body, where it gives energy and life itself.

Within every cell in the body is a furnace called the *mitochondria*. Imagine yourself in front of a crackling, warm fire. It burns safely and quietly most of the time. But on occasion, out flies a cinder that lands on your carpet, burning a little hole in it. One cinder by itself does not pose much of a threat; but if this sparking and popping continues month after month, year after year, you will end up with a pretty ragged carpet in front of your fireplace.

Similarly, this microscopic organism, the mitochondria, within the cell reduces oxygen by the transfer of electrons to create energy into the form of

ATP,[1] and produces a by-product of water. This process goes on without a hitch at least 98 percent of the time. But the full complement of four electrons needed to reduce oxygen to water does not always happen as planned and a "free radical" is produced.

Chemical Pathway for Oxygen Reduction to Water

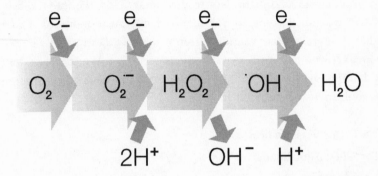

The cinder from the fireplace represents a free radical, and the carpet represents your body. Whichever part of the body receives the most free radical damage is the first to wear out and potentially develop degenerative disease. If it is your eyes, you could develop macular degeneration or cataracts. If it is your blood vessels, you could have a heart attack or a stroke. If it is your joint space, you could develop arthritis. If it is your brain, you could develop Alzheimer's or Parkinson's disease. After the passing of time, our bodies can look just like the carpet in front of the fireplace: pretty ratty.

Together we have just imagined the "bright" side of oxygen and the life it brings (like the warmth of the fire), but we cannot deny the rest of the story. This is the part many of us have never heard about: the demise that unruly free radicals causes, otherwise known as *oxidative stress.*

This oxidative stress is the underlying cause of almost all of these chronic degenerative diseases. Though this occurs on the inside, it is much easier to observe the oxidative stress that is occurring on the outside surface of the body, the skin. Have you ever seen a several-generation family portrait? If you looked closely at their skin, you would see the significant difference between that of the youngest family member and the oldest. The effect you see is due to oxidative stress of the skin. This same decay is happening inside our bodies too.

The Dark Side of Oxygen

As I said, through biochemical research we are learning that the underlying cause of degenerative disease, and possibly the aging process itself, is oxidative stress that free radicals cause.

Chemically, the violent action of these free radicals has been shown to actually produce bursts of light. Not readily neutralized, the free radicals set off a chain reaction leading to potentially dangerous conditions. Did you know there is literally a war waging within your body? During the silent, day-to-day breakdown of oxygen, a vital battle is occurring. We can consider this war by defining the specific roles of its fascinating and clear-cut characters in the metabolism of our body:

> *The Enemy*: Free Radicals
>
> *The Allies*: Antioxidants
>
> *Behind the Lines*: Supporting Nutrients—the B cofactors (B1, B2, B6, B12, and folic acid) and antioxidant minerals. These are like the supply lines of fuel, bullets, and food and the mechanics who keep the machines running in combat situations.
>
> *Enemy Reinforcement:* Conditions that increase the number of free radicals that the body produces, such as pollutants in our air, food, and water; excessive stress, poor exercise habits, and so on.
>
> *MASH*: Repair unit for the injured Free Radicals.

Free radicals are mainly oxygen molecules or atoms that have at least one unpaired electron in their outer orbit. In the process of utilizing oxygen during normal metabolism within the cell to create energy (called oxidation), active free oxygen radicals are created. They essentially have an electrical charge and desire to try to get an electron from any molecule or substance in the vicinity. They have such violent movement that they have been shown chemically to create bursts of light within the body. If these free radicals are not rapidly neutralized by an antioxidant, they may create even more volatile free radicals or cause damage to the cell membrane, vessel wall, proteins, fats, or even the DNA nucleus of the cell.[2] Scientific and medical literature refers to this damage as oxidative stress.

Our Ally: Antioxidants

God did not leave us defenseless against the onslaught of free radicals. In fact, when I look at the intricate complexity of our antioxidant defense system, I have great appreciation of how marvelously and wonderfully we are made. We actually have our own army of antioxidants, which are able to neutralize free radicals and render them harmless. Antioxidants are like the glass doors or a fine-wired mesh screen that we place in front of the fireplace. The sparks (free radicals) are still going to fly; however, your carpet (your body) is protected.

An antioxidant is any substance that has the ability to give up an electron to a free radical and balance out the unpaired electron, which neutralizes the free radical. Our body even has the ability to create some of its own antioxidants. In fact the body produces three major antioxidant defense systems: the superoxide dismutase, catalase, and glutathione peroxidase. It is not important that you remember these names, but it is important to realize that we do have a natural antioxidant defense system.

Our bodies do not produce all the antioxidants we need, however. The rest of our antioxidants must come from food or, as you will learn, nutritional supplementation. As long as adequate amounts of antioxidants are available for the amount of free radicals produced, no damage is wrought to our bodies. But when more free radicals are produced than there are antioxidants available, oxidative stress occurs. When this situation persists for a prolonged period of time, we can develop a chronic degenerative disease and begin to lose the war within.

Balance is the key to winning this ongoing war. We must keep the offensive and defensive equally matched. In order to win our bodies must always be armed with more antioxidants than free radicals.

Most antioxidants we get from vegetables and fruits. The most common antioxidants are vitamin C, vitamin E, vitamin A, and beta-carotene. We can obtain numerous other antioxidants from our food; these include coenzyme Q10, alpha-lipoic acid, and the colorful bioflavanoid antioxidants. It is important to realize that antioxidants work in synergy with one another to disarm free radicals in different areas of the body. Like the varied positions of military defense, these antioxidants each have specific roles. Some antioxidants have the ability to actually regenerate other antioxidants so they can neutralize more free radicals. For example, vitamin C is water-soluble and is therefore the best antioxidant to target free radicals within the blood and plasma. Vitamin E is fat-soluble and is the best antioxidant within the cell membrane. Glutathione is the best antioxidant within the cell itself. Alpha-lipoic acid works both within the cell membrane and the plasma. Vitamin C and alpha-lipoic acid have the ability to regenerate vitamin E and glutathione so they can be used again.

The more antioxidants, the merrier! Our goal is to have more than enough antioxidants to neutralize the free radicals we produce. This can occur only when a complete and balanced army of antioxidants is available at all times.

Behind the Lines

Every army needs a support system behind the battle lines—this is critical in the final outcome of a war. Simply having adequate amounts of antioxidants (or soldiers) available to neutralize the free radicals we produce is not the complete answer. Soldiers need continual supplies—ammunition, food, water, and clothing—if they are going to perform at their peak level.

Antioxidant soldiers need the availability of other nutrients in *adequate* amounts to fulfill their duty on the front lines against the threat of free radicals. They need sufficient antioxidant minerals such as copper, zinc, manganese, and selenium, which aid in the chemical reactions of the antioxidants so they are able to do their job effectively. If enough of these minerals are not available, oxidative stress will usually occur.

Antioxidants also need certain cofactors in their enzymatic reactions in order to perform their job properly. Cofactors are the military support system, like the mechanics or supply officers, fuel tanks, and makers of the ammunition. These are primarily the B cofactors: folic acid, vitamins B1, B2, B6, and B12. We need a good store of both the antioxidant minerals and cofactors if we are going to have any hope of winning the war within.

The battleground is actually more complicated than I have just described. You see, the number of free radicals we produce is never constant. The production of free radicals varies in the daily process of normal metabolism and reduction of oxygen, and our defense system never knows exactly how many free radicals it will have to deal with on any given day. Many factors may increase the amount of free radicals we produce and in turn must neutralize.

What causes the production of more free radicals than our bodies can fight off? This question drove me to hours and hours of research. I learned to look at the different sources of free radicals to find the answer. Let us now discuss those culprits.

What Creates Free Radicals

Excessive Exercise

In *The Antioxidant Revolution*, Dr. Kenneth Cooper emphasized the fact that excessive exercise can significantly increase the amount of free radicals our body produces. Dr. Cooper became quite concerned when he saw several strenuous exercisers die prematurely of heart attacks, strokes, and cancer. These were individuals who may have run thirty or forty marathons in their lifetimes while at the same time having lengthy daily workouts.

During his research for the antioxidant book, Dr. Cooper realized the potential harm that overexercising could bring. When we exercise mildly or moderately, the numbers of free radicals you and I produce go up only slightly. In contrast, when we exercise excessively, the numbers of free radicals we produce go off the graph, increasing exponentially.

The Antioxidant Revolution concludes by warning readers that excessive exercise can actually be harmful to our health, especially if we continue it over several years. Dr. Cooper recommends a moderate exercise program for everyone, but he also suggests that everyone take antioxidants in supplementation. Only serious athletes should undertake strenuous exercise, and they should balance it with significant amounts of antioxidant supplements.[3]

Excessive Stress

As with exercise, a mild to moderate amount of emotional stress produces only a slight increase in free radicals. Severe emotional stress, however, causes the number of free radicals to rise significantly, creating oxidative stress. Have you ever noticed that when you are under a lot of pressure you frequently become sick? How many times have you known a close friend or family member who has been under tremendous stress for a prolonged period of time only to discover he has developed cancer or had a first heart attack?

I don't have many patients who have run multiple marathons in their lifetimes, but I have hundreds of patients who are under prolonged emotional stress. Financial, work, and personal pressures have so complicated our lives that emotional stress is the most pressing health factor I deal with in my practice. Once you begin to understand the seriousness of oxidative stress, you begin to appreciate the dangerous effects of long-term emotional pressure on your health, and you can begin to counteract it.

Air Pollution

The environment has a tremendous influence on the amount of free radicals our bodies produces. Air pollution is a major cause of oxidative stress in our lungs and in our bodies. When you drive into any major city today, you not only can see the thick haze, you can taste it.

I remember my medical-school days at the University of Colorado Medical School in 1970. During my rotation on the neurology unit, I had to make rounds at 6:00 A.M. Before I started, I would walk down to the west windows and admire the sunrise reflecting its light on the beautiful Rocky Mountains. I then quickly began my rounds, which took about two hours each day. When I finished, I would run back to that beautiful view of the mountains before my first clinical lecture. To my amazement, I usually could not even see the mountains by then. All I could see were some white outlines through the thick, red haze. What a dramatic change occurred during the two hours people commuted to their jobs.

The health effects of air pollution have caused significant concern. Air pollution contains ozone, nitrogen dioxide, sulfur dioxide, and several hydrocarbon molecules, all of which generate a significant amount of free radicals. When you are exposed to these toxins day in and day out, they have a major effect on your health. Air pollution has been implicated in the causes of asthma, chronic bronchitis, heart attacks, and even cancer. Understanding oxidative stress as the underlying cause of all of these diseases allows us to develop a strategy of protecting ourselves from the damaging effects of air pollution.

We must consider another aspect of air pollution: the occupational exposure to mineral dust such as asbestos fibers. The addition of iron-containing fibers in asbestos can generate even more free radicals. Long-term exposure has been shown to cause lung cancer and interstitial fibrosis (a serious scarring of the lung). There are many other occupational hazards: Farmers are exposed to the fine dust in their barns and grain bins. Industrial workers are exposed to various chemicals and fine dust in their work.

Needless to say, the quality of the air we breathe is a major health consideration.

Cigarette Smoke

One might anticipate that smog or chemicals pose the biggest threat to our health on a daily basis. But would you believe the greatest cause of oxidative stress in our bodies is cigarette and cigar smoke? It's true. Smoking has been associated with the increased risk of asthma, emphysema, chronic bronchitis, lung cancer, and cardiovascular disease. We all are aware of the health consequences of smoking, but it is fascinating to realize that the underlying problem is the amount of oxidative stress smoking produces in our bodies. Cigarette smoke contains several different toxins, all of which increase the amount of free radicals appearing not only in our lungs but also throughout our bodies. No other habit or addiction affects our overall health more dramatically than smoking.

I know of nothing more addictive than nicotine. When Dr. C. Everett Koop, the U.S. surgeon general, called smoking an addiction rather than a habit, he forever changed the way we look at smoking.[4] How? He informed the public about the addictive qualities of nicotine, which the tobacco companies supposedly had known about for half a century. In fact strong evidence exists that says you can become addicted to nicotine within two to three weeks.[5] Is it any wonder that it is so difficult for people to quit smoking? I have found it much more difficult for patients to stop smoking than to stop drinking alcohol. I believe the absurd and far-reaching cost to our health that cigarette smoke causes is far more than we can determine.

What about secondary smoke? Medical research now proves that individuals who are exposed to significant secondary smoke have an increased risk of asthma, emphysema, heart attacks, and even lung cancer.[6] This is the reason so many laws have been passed restricting cigarette smoke in public places.

Have you recently been exposed to a group of people smoking in a confined area? I recall driving my daughter back from college this past month. I had to stop in a small town to fill up the car with gas. When I walked into the station to pay for the gas, six local residents were sitting around a small table, all smoking cigarettes as they sipped coffee. I could hardly take a breath without coughing. I actually began to feel sick. For those who are not accustomed to cigarette smoke, its effects are more clearly recognizable. I am sure there are times and situations that you've had similar experiences. It doesn't take much imagination to realize that if you are exposed to secondary smoke on a daily basis, it will have a major impact on your health.

Pollution of Our Food and Water

Are you thirsty? In 1988 the U.S. Department of Public Health warned us that 85 percent of American drinking water is contaminated. And I can hardly believe things have gotten better over the past decade. More than fifty thousand different chemicals now contaminate our water supplies. Here's a frightening fact: the average water treatment plant can test for only thirty to forty of these chemicals. In addition heavy metals such as lead, cadmium, and aluminum contaminate most of our water supplies. More than fifty-five thousand regulated chemical dumps in America, in addition to the estimated two hundred thousand unregulated chemical dumps, are leaking into the water tables across the nation. When we ingest this contaminated water, the production of free radicals increases significantly.[7]

Americans have resorted to drinking bottled, filtered, and distilled water in unprecedented amounts today. But you should know this: except for distilled water, you have no way of knowing the quality of the water you are paying so dearly for since it is an entirely unregulated market.

Since the Second World War, more than sixty thousand new chemicals have been introduced into our environment. No less than one thousand new-fangled chemicals are introduced to our environment each year. Herbicides, pesticides, and fungicides are used in the production of most of our foods. Medical research has shown us that all of these chemicals create increased oxidative stress when we consume them. Some are more dangerous than others, but they all have potential health risks. These chemicals have allowed our food industry to produce the most abundant food supply ever known. But what is the cost to our health?

Ultraviolet Sunlight

It is a known fact that people get two-thirds of their lifetime sun exposure to their skin prior to their twentieth birthday. This means you, the reader of this book, have most likely already exposed your skin to the sun's damaging ultraviolet rays.

Several different studies have shown ultraviolet light to produce increased free radicals in human skin.[8] This in turn has been proven to produce damage to the DNA in the cells of our skin, which leads to skin cancer. These studies provide the best direct evidence that oxidative stress leads to the development of cancer.

UVB light is the primary culprit responsible for the sun's burning rays, but both UVA and UVB light increase free-radical production in the skin and thus oxidative stress in the skin. When you apply your favorite sunscreen, which contains an SPF rating of thirty or greater, you are protecting yourself primarily against UVB light. This allows us to stay out in the sun longer because we are not getting sunburned. But these sunscreens do not offer much, if any, protection against UVA light, which creates significantly more free radicals deeper into the skin. This may in part explain why we have seen a fivefold increase in almost every skin cancer over the past twenty years.

We are finally seeing sunscreens on the market that offer protection against both UVA and UVB sunlight. Obviously, this is the kind of sunscreen you want to purchase to protect yourself and your children against both being sunburned and developing skin cancer. I would encourage everyone to keep a watchful eye on his skin for any unusual growths or changes in pigmented moles.

Medications and Radiation

Every medication I prescribe causes increased oxidative stress in the body. Chemotherapeutic drugs and radiation therapy primarily work by creating oxidative stress damage to the cancer cells, which kills them. This is the main reason patients find these drugs and therapies so hard to tolerate. The increased oxidative stress also causes collateral damage to normal cells.

It is important to remember that every drug is essentially a foreign substance to the body, and the body has to work harder trying to metabolize and eliminate it. This puts increased demand on many of the metabolic pathways in the liver and the body as a whole. Thus increased production of free radicals takes place and the potential to create oxidative stress grows.

The industrialized world of the twenty-first century has become overdependent on medications. The consumption of medications in the U.S. and in the world is obviously at an all-time high. Even though every drug has been tested to show it provides a benefit, each also carries an inherent risk. Serious adverse drug reactions are the fourth leading cause of death in the United States. It's true: properly prescribed and administered medications are responsible for more than one hundred thousand deaths, and two million hospital admissions, in the U.S. each year.[9] Much of the inherent risk of medications is due to the oxidative stress these drugs can potentially produce.

•   •   •

More than seventy chronic degenerative diseases are the direct result of the "toxic" effects of oxygen. In other words the root cause of these diseases is oxidative stress. Medical science has now shown us that the underlying cause of these terrible diseases we all fear with the coming of age is the unsuspected dark side of oxygen.

If you have ever restored an old car, you have encountered the detrimental effects of rust. It can weaken and disintegrate one of the earth's strongest materials: metal. And like an abandoned vehicle out in a field, our bodies literally begin to rust if they are not protected. A slow corrosion begins in our body and, like a weak spot in metal, whichever part of the body wears out first will determine what type of degenerative disease we may develop.

Fortunately, not only do our bodies possess a tremendous antioxidant defense system; they also possess a remarkable repair system. The next chapter explains how this MASH unit is able to repair the inevitable casualties of the war that is raging within every cell in our bodies.

PART II

WINNING THE WAR WITHIN

FOUR | Our Repair System: The MASH Unit

THERE WILL ALWAYS BE CASUALTIES OF WAR. AND THE WAR THAT IS being waged in our bodies is no different. In spite of our tremendous antioxidant defense systems, the enemy gets through and damages lipids (fats), proteins, cell walls, vessel walls, and even the DNA nucleus of the cell. Many research centers have now confirmed the existence of damage removal and repair systems for all of these oxidized (damaged by free radicals) proteins, cell wall lipids, and DNA. Simply put, our bodies have a sophisticated, state-of-the-art MASH unit.[1]

When I was a young physician, I realized the strong possibility that I would be called up to be part of a MASH unit in the Vietnam War. During my training at the University of Colorado Medical School, most of the residents had been to Vietnam and most of the interns were on their way. But as it turned out, by the time I finished my internship the war had pretty much ended and the draft was no longer in effect.

Though I never actually went to Vietnam, I remember the original movie, *M*A*S*H*, with all of the wounded soldiers being brought in by helicopter. The stressful, frantic surgeries that followed in attempts to mend soldiers are still vivid in my mind. Did you know this same scenario is happening every day inside our bodies? We have a sophisticated team of triage nurses, anesthesiologists, and surgeons that are busy repairing the damage caused by the free radicals our body is producing.

There is both a direct repair system and an indirect repair system within each of our bodies. We really don't know much about the direct repair system; however, it is well documented that it does exist. Most of our knowledge centers instead on the indirect repair system.

In the health care field, triage nurses are the ones who evaluate the patient to determine which patient is in the most critical condition and will be seen by the doctor first. Extensive studies have revealed that the "triage nurses" in our bodies recognize damaged cell parts and then repair them.[2] The body doesn't just patch these cells; it actually tears them down completely and then rebuilds from scratch. Incredible, isn't it? Damaged proteins become brand-new proteins, made with recycled amino acids. The body repairs altered fats and DNA in a similar matter. It is critical that you understand that the body has an amazing built-in ability to heal itself.

As I reflect on the complex nature of this repair system and the functions of the cell, I know beyond doubt this is no random act of nature. During my first year of medical school, I studied the anatomy and function of the eye. As I observed the intricacy of the structure, I realized that this object could never have been the result of accidental chance and random selection. The retina itself is made up of twelve intricate layers and billions of specialized cells. The rods and cones in the retina gather the light waves and send these messages to the brain. Our brain interprets these impulses and creates our vision in vivid, moving, full color. Just take a moment to look out your nearest window and simply marvel at the gift of sight. This is no accident—it is an ingenious creation!

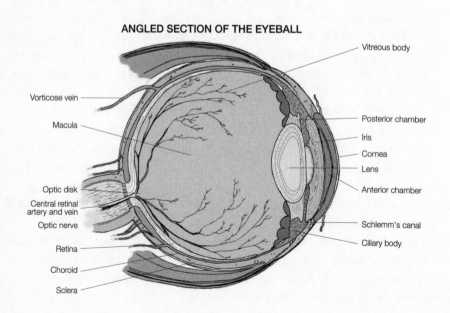

ANGLED SECTION OF THE EYEBALL

Vitreous body

Vorticose vein

Macula

Posterior chamber

Iris

Cornea

Lens

Optic disk

Anterior chamber

Central retinal artery and vein

Optic nerve

Schlemm's canal

Ciliary body

Retina

Choroid

Sclera

These same thoughts come back to me now as I study the body's astonishing immune system and antioxidant defense system. I have no doubt that God is our true Healer. "I will give thanks to Thee, for I am fearfully and wonderfully made," David exclaimed.[3] God created a magnificent "earth suit" for us to take care of and to nurture. The *best* defense against getting chronic degenerative diseases is provided in our own bodies, not in the drugs I prescribe.

Biochemical researchers are now able to study the inner workings and complexities of each cell in our body. The cell is not simply a shell that contains a soft consistent gel, as many early evolutionists believed. It is instead filled with sophisticated structures, genetic codes, and transport systems that support life by their elaborate biochemical reactions.

When I look at an ink pen, I try to imagine that some plastic, metal, and ink sat around for millions and millions of years and then suddenly, by chance, accidentally formed this pen. But then I think, *Maybe someone made it!* The human body is a profoundly complicated creation, and the secrets we are learning about how it works and functions make it all the more incredible.

The Devastation of War

In spite of this tremendous defense and repair system inherent in our bodies, damage can still occur. Oxidative stress has the potential to overpower all of these protective systems and cause chronic degenerative diseases. During periods of particularly high production of free radicals, the defense and repair system can break down and no longer cope with the number of damaged proteins, fats, cell membranes, and DNA structures.

When not properly repaired, damaged proteins can create further problems in cell function. Damaged lipids lead to rigid cell membranes; oxidized cholesterol often leads to hardening of the arteries. And poorly repaired DNA chains lead to cell mutation as implicated in cancer and aging.

Simply stated, when we overwork our built-in antioxidant defense and repair systems, significant damage occurs to the body and eventually may lead to any one of a number of chronic degenerative diseases. Biochemical researchers realized years ago that based on their estimates of damaged cells from oxidative stress, we would die quickly from this damage to vital cellular parts if the antioxidant enzymes and compounds were our only means of protection.[4] This is why it is essential that we optimize all of these natural defense systems.

Our Best Defense

Outside of Eden, our food and our environment have totally changed. Consequently, our bodies are literally under attack. Air and water pollution, the long-range effects of smoking, and a faster-paced and pressure-packed lifestyle add up to stress on our bodies. Even our diet has suffered. Our food supply is significantly deficient in quality nutrients. In 1970 Americans spent about $6 billion on fast food; in 2000 they spent more than $110 billion. Americans now spend more money on fast food than on higher education, personal computers, computer software, or new cars. They spend more on fast food than on movies, books, magazines, newspapers, videos, and recorded music combined.[5]

All of these factors mean free radicals are more active and damaging than ever. Nutritional medicine, supplementing our diet with vital antioxidant vitamins and minerals, is the only means we have to supercharge our body's natural defense and immune system.

Nutritional medicine protects our health by enhancing the natural defense systems God has created for a polluted world. When we provide the proper nutrients at the optimal levels that the body needs to function, it can do what God intended.

Once you understand the concept of oxidative stress and its deleterious effect on your body, you will want to learn how to have victory over it. You will want to know how to have enough antioxidants and their supporting nutrients on board to handle the number of free radicals your body produces.

As simple as this sounds, it is a revolutionary concept when it comes to our health. The longer we are able to prevent or delay these chronic degenerative diseases, the longer we are able to enjoy good health. We are all going to die sometime, unless the Lord returns first, but as my friend claimed, I too want to live until I die.

Balance Is the Goal

When I was a young teenager, the federal government decided to take most of the silver out of our coins. Instantly, all the old coins, which were solid silver, were worth much more than the new coins the government was minting. Many individuals and businesses began buying up these solid silver coins and, of course, we teens gathered up as many solid silver coins as we could find too.

I was especially in luck. My dad owned a Dairy Queen, and he brought home a pile of coins each night that I would have to roll up in paper rolls. I would carefully select out the solid silver coins (with my dad's permission) and then take them out to sell them.

I loved pulling open the heavy wooden door at the hardware store off of Main Street. The musty smells of old wood, furniture polish, and oil would welcome me along with the friendly voice of Mr. Smalley saying, "Hello there, son!" When Mr. Smalley saw me coming he'd bring out a scale to weigh my coins (he paid by the weight). He used the old-fashioned kind that had two trays on either side of a balance arm. Mr. Smalley loaded my coins on one tray, then placed weights, one at a time, onto the other tray.

I remember holding my breath with excitement when he had to keep pulling out more and more brass weights to counterbalance all my coins. As it got close, he'd glance over at me out from under the bill of his cap and wink. "Bingo!" he'd say when the scale finally balanced out. Then he'd tell me how much money I was going to get for all those silver coins.

Balance is key when it comes to oxidative stress. The anecdote I've told offers a useful analogy. Our body is always trying to put enough brass weights (antioxidants) on one tray to balance out all of the silver coins (free radicals). The body makes some of those antioxidants, but they are simply not enough. Our food, especially fruits and vegetables, used to provide all the extra antioxidants our bodies needed. A generation or two ago, people ate more whole, fresh foods that contain significantly more antioxidants than today's diet does. But as a result of the tremendous increase in the toxins in our environment today, along with the depleted nutrients we receive from our highly processed foods, our scale is out of balance—in favor of the silver coins (free radicals).

We need to add nutritional supplements to the balance in order to provide the level of antioxidants our bodies need. In fact we want the brass weights to tip the scale in its favor because then we won't have oxidative stress.

Remember, there are two sides of the coin: the amount of free radicals our bodies have to deal with and an optimized antioxidant/repair system. In the chapters that follow, I will lay out the medical evidence that shows how you as an individual can improve your antioxidant defense system by eating a healthy diet, exercising moderately, and taking high-quality nutritional supplements. I will also show you how, by taking what I refer to as "optimizers" (super potent antioxidants), you can even regain your health if you have already lost it.

First, meet someone who learned firsthand how powerful nutritional medicine can be.

Evelyn's Story

Evelyn had just moved to Spokane, Washington, with her family when a serious automobile accident left her hospitalized with multiple injuries. Her left side became weak and numb, and the doctors were worried she had suffered a stroke. Test after heartrending test left her and her family in the dark. They had no idea what was happening to her body.

Approximately six months later, during which time Evelyn saw eighteen different physicians, she was diagnosed with multiple sclerosis. One of the great causes of oxidative stress is injuries or major surgeries, and Evelyn's physicians felt that the trauma of the accident had triggered the MS.

Evelyn has always tried to have a good attitude toward her diagnosis and promised never to let the disease get her down. Doctors started her on a drug called Betaseron, which is a common drug used for MS. Betaserone is actually beta interferon, a chemical that tries to build up the immune system—very expensive and very hard to tolerate. Evelyn's body was just barely able to tolerate this medication, and she became very sick. After two months she told her family and her doctor she would not continue taking the drug. Her family was supportive, realizing that the terrible side effects were not worth any gain she might receive.

"I was devastated and spent many days depressed," Evelyn remembers. "I would stare out my window and ask those haunting questions: *Why me?* and *Why now?* I spent nights wandering the halls of our home or sitting at our parlor window crying. It was my only time to be alone, when I could express my deepest emotions."

Evelyn attended support group meetings with her husband and children. She and her family began making adjustments to their lifestyle in order to accommodate and care for her needs. Evelyn also faced the possibility of sudden blindness, a symptom of MS that some people experience. "I would sit at the foot of my children's beds," she recalls, "watching them sleep, memorizing their faces, the color of their hair, their peaceful expressions so I wouldn't forget what they looked like. I would write in my journal and try to document everything I could remember about my children. A day didn't pass that I would take a single moment for granted."

It was not long before Evelyn began to decline. Over the next four years, she continued to lose strength in both of her legs, and eventually in her arms and hands. She had to use a four-pronged cane for a while; a few months later she needed a walker. Even more frustrating and discouraging was the fact that she began to experience bowel and bladder retention. This not only made her feel uncomfortable, it also led to several bladder and kidney infections. She became totally dependent on her family for both her physical and emotional needs.

Through it all Evelyn's attitude was amazing. She could hardly move or go anywhere without the help of her walker or family. She could see the shock at her decline written all over her friends' faces. But Evelyn didn't give up. In response to her disease, this wife and mom started physical therapy and began to research MS on her own.

Evelyn tried some alternative therapies but continued to decline. Then, almost four years after her diagnosis, she decided to try taking potent nutritional supplements in an attempt to slow down the progression of her disease. She started with some strong antioxidant and mineral tablets along with grape-seed extract and a natural nutrient called *Coenzyme Q10*. Within weeks Evelyn began to feel better.

"For the first time in years, I slept through the night and woke up feeling rested," she reports. "I no longer needed a nap during the day, and I didn't have bladder or bowel problems. I experienced an increase in my endurance level. My strength began returning in my legs and my arms. I could even run up the stairs to answer the phone, which stunned my children. In fact I completely surprised my daughter, Tasha, when I started to jump rope with her. For the first time in a long time, I was able to walk outside barefoot and feel the grass under my toes."

Evelyn had many other surprises as she continued taking her nutritional supplements. For one, even before the accident, she had suffered from heart palpitations. Along with the improvement she noticed in her MS, she also realized that her heart was beating again normally. When she approached her doctor about the possibility of quitting the drug, Norpace, that controlled her heart arrhythmia, he did some testing and wrote on her chart, "Off all meds." Evelyn's life had been miraculously changed.

What happened? Why did Evelyn improve so much? At the time I became involved with Evelyn I had never seen anyone with MS experience such results. I had witnessed many patients with flare-ups from their disease going into remission. But their overall strength and body function still slowly declined. Evelyn's story was markedly different.

By applying the principles you will learn in this book, Evelyn was able to win the war within. She began providing enough antioxidants and their supporting nutrients to restore balance to her body and bring the oxidative stress back under control. She built up her body's natural immune system while improving her body's natural repair system.

I'm happy to report that Evelyn has continued to improve and now leads an active life. It has been more than seven years since she started her nutritional program. She still has MS, of course, and has to be careful. But she is living life to the fullest. She continues to go to her MS support group—not for herself but to encourage others.

Evelyn's neurologist still does not know what to think about her miraculous turnaround. He recently ordered a repeat MRI of her brain. To his amazement, the white plaque spread throughout the brain that is so diagnostic of MS had significantly diminished. This could mean only one thing: healing had occurred during the interim. Normally, these typical lesions on the brain only increase in number. Needless to say, Evelyn's neurologist was speechless.

Here is strong evidence that the body is still able to heal itself when necessary nutrients are available at optimal levels. Evelyn's story is just one illustration of the benefits of winning the war within.

●   ●   ●

You now understand the basic concept of oxidative stress. So you now need to take a closer look at each of these individual chronic degenerative diseases to better understand how you can best prevent them. If you already have a serious degenerative disease, you will discover how you can best redeem your health. You will discover the wondrous results of a whole new approach of preventive medicine: cellular nutrition.

FIVE | Heart Disease: An Inflammatory Disease

DAILY YOU AND I HEAR REMINDERS ABOUT THE SERIOUSNESS OF America's cholesterol problem. And as I mentioned in Chapter 2, heart disease is the number-one cause of death in the United States. Like me, you probably assume what such statistics and much of the media suggest: cholesterol is the cause of heart disease.

If so, you may be as stunned as I was to learn that cholesterol is not the culprit behind heart disease; the inflammation of blood vessels is. My research revealed that more than half of heart-attack patients in the United States have normal cholesterol levels![1] And can you guess what I discovered significantly reduces, or eliminates entirely, inflammation of the blood vessels? That's right: nutritional supplements.

This finding is revolutionary to the treatment and prevention of heart attacks. Rather than concentrating only on lowering cholesterol, you need to understand the necessary steps to decreasing the cause of the inflammation in your arteries. This approach could have significant and dramatic implications in the prevention and reversal of heart disease.

What About Cholesterol?

Did you know that elevated cholesterol in the blood was not always considered a risk factor for coronary artery disease and stroke? When I first began practicing medicine in 1972, we considered any cholesterol level less than 320 normal. I distinctly remember telling patients who had a cholesterol level of 280 or 310 not to worry because their cholesterol levels were normal.

It really wasn't until the late seventies that we began to realize the higher the cholesterol levels, the greater the risk of developing a heart attack or stroke. This was based in large part on the Framingham studies, which followed a large population of patients who lived in Framingham, Massachusetts. Scientists noted in these studies that as the cholesterol levels increased, so did the frequency of heart attacks. Following this research, cholesterol levels greater than 200 were considered abnormal and a cholesterol level greater than 240 placed the patient at high risk of developing a heart attack.[2]

In the early 1980s physicians began to learn that not all cholesterol was bad. We learned that HDL (high density lipoproteins) cholesterol is actually good, and the higher our HDL cholesterol is, the better. It is the LDL (low density lipoproteins) cholesterol that is bad. LDL cholesterol accumulates along the artery walls, forming plaque and narrowing the arteries. The HDL cholesterol actually comes along and cleans up the artery.

After this discovery we started checking not only total cholesterol levels but also determining the amounts of both good and bad cholesterol present. We calculate a ratio by dividing the total cholesterol by the HDL cholesterol. The lower this ratio is, the better off the patient is when it comes to heart disease. It is now common practice to routinely check both HDL and LDL cholesterol levels. Needless to say, we are all acutely aware of the importance of cholesterol and the detrimental effects of LDL cholesterol.

What I have shared with you so far is pretty common knowledge. Are you ready for the uncommon knowledge?

LDL cholesterol is really not "bad." God didn't make a mistake when He created it. Native LDL cholesterol, the kind that the body originally makes, is good. In fact it is essential for building good cell membranes, other cell parts, and many different hormones that our bodies need. We could not live without it. In fact if we don't get enough from our diet, our bodies will actually make this form of cholesterol.

Problems begin to occur only when free radicals change or oxidize native LDL cholesterol. It is this modified LDL cholesterol that is truly "bad." In a 1989 issue of the *New England Journal of Medicine*, Dr. Daniel Steinberg postulated that if patients had adequate antioxidants on board to quell oxidization, the LDL cholesterol would not become bad.[3]

In the years since Dr. Steinberg's theory was released, hundreds of studies have been conducted in an attempt to either prove or disprove his theory.

You can appreciate why scientists and researchers met Dr. Steinberg's new theory with such enthusiasm. After all, of the approximately 1.5 million heart attacks in the United States this year alone, almost half of these patients will be under the age of sixty-five.[4] We have all known friends or loved ones who seemed to be in excellent health only to find out that they have died suddenly of a heart attack. If Steinberg's theory turned out to be true, doors would open wide to a vast array of new preventive and treatment protocols.

In 1997 researcher Dr. Marco Diaz made an impressive review of all of the studies that had appeared in mainline medical journals since Dr. Steinberg had first presented his theory. Diaz concluded that patients with the highest levels of antioxidants in their bodies indeed had the least amount of coronary artery disease.[5]

Animal studies done during this time also supported Dr. Steinberg's theory.[6] Antioxidants and their supporting nutrients have become the new hope in the war against our number-one killer: heart disease.

The Nature of the Inflammatory Response

LDL cholesterol isn't the only instigator behind inflammation of the blood vessels. Other main causes include something called *homocysteine* (which I'll discuss in Chapter 6) and the free radicals that cigarette smoking, hypertension, fatty foods, and diabetes cause.

The inflammation that takes place in our arteries is quite similar to the inflammatory reactions found elsewhere in the body. I will attempt to explain this process in lay terms so that you will have a better understanding of what is actually taking place on a cellular level. Don't get caught up in trying to understand the minute details of this process. (This is difficult even for most physicians to understand, so don't feel bad if you are not getting all of it.) I will then explain how you can best protect yourself against this insult to your arteries—it is really quite simple.

When you look at the cross section of a typical, medium-sized artery (Figure 1) you simply need to look at the first layer of cells called the *endothelium*. This is the tissue-thin lining of the artery. Everything that I am going to talk about involves this thin layer of cells and the area just under the lining's surface called the *subendothelial space* (see Figure 2).

Figure 1 — Normal Artery

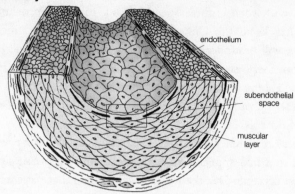

The inner surface of the artery is made up of a sensitive, single layer of cells called the endothelium and underneath is the muscular layer. Between the endothelium and the muscular layer is the subendothelial space. This is where all the damage begins to take place.

Figure 2 — Oxidation of LDL Cholesterol

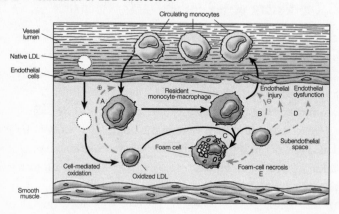

The native LDL cholesterol actually becomes trapped in the subendothelial space where it can be easily oxidized if there are not adequate antioxidants available. This oxidized LDL cholesterol is then easily "gobbled up" by the monocyte white cells until it is literally "stuffed" with fat. Remember, this does not happen if the LDL cholesterol is not oxidized. When this monocyte becomes stuffed with the oxidized LDL cholesterol, it becomes a "Foam-cell." The Foam-cell then causes damage to the sensitive lining of the artery by creating oxidative stress in this area. This leads to injury and dysfunction of the endothelium, and the process of hardening of the arteries is off and running.

The inflammatory response is a four-step process.

Step 1: The Initial Insult to the Endothelium

The endothelium is an extremely sensitive lining that is vulnerable to even the slightest irritation. Almost all research scientists now believe that hardening of the arteries begins when oxidative stress damages or irritates this single cell layer.

Oxidized LDL cholesterol, homocysteine, and excessive free radicals cause the oxidative stress that *injures* the endothelium. This occurs when native LDL cholesterol is able to pass into the area just beneath the lining of the artery (called the subendothelial space) where it becomes oxidized. This cholesterol then begins to irritate the lining of the artery.

Step 2: Inflammatory Response

Our body has a defense system designed to protect this endothelium of the artery. In the event of injury, our body responds by sending in certain white cells (mainly monocytes) in an attempt to eliminate the harmful oxidized LDL cholesterol. Here the defense team of monocytes starts gobbling up the enemy in an attempt to minimize the irritation to the endothelium. If this inflammatory response is successful, the problem is over and the lining of the artery will be repaired. But this is not what usually happens.

Think of a monocyte as a white minivan. As it drives around, picking up children and letting them off in their proper places, it is limited to the number of children it can carry at any one time because it has only so many seats and seat belts. On a good day the same is true for monocytes. When we're healthy they zoom around, picking up native LDL cholesterol and dropping off other native LDL cholesterol. And just like a minivan, monocytes can carry only so many native LDL cholesterol particles at a time. This is known as a *natural feedback mechanism*.

When native LDL cholesterol becomes oxidized, the cholesterol particles are no longer harmless little children. Instead, they now pose a threat to the body, and the monocytes pick them up via a totally different method. Monocytes continue to gather the delinquent oxidized LDL cells, but they don't let any out. This would be like a gang of severely obese juveniles clamoring into the minivan through the rear door without its driver having any control whatsoever on the number of kids getting in. If this were to happen, the van would be immobilized and soon begin to jam up traffic.

When the monocyte encounters bad cholesterol, it is in a similar fix. Because there is no natural feedback mechanism, the monocyte gets crammed so full of oxidized LDL cholesterol (fat) that it becomes a foam cell. This is just like what you are picturing in your mind: it is a cell that looks like a ball of fat. This foam cell then attaches itself to the lining of the artery and eventually forms the initial defect of hardening of the arteries, which is called a *fatty streak*.

The fatty streak is an inflammatory lesion. It is the initial step in this process called *atherosclerosis*. If the process would simply stop here, the body would at least have a chance to clear this defect. But this is not the case. As in any war, this process has some collateral damage. In other words the thin, vulnerable layer of cells lining our arteries is damaged even more by the very process that is supposed to heal it. This actually creates more inflammation, which attracts more monocytes and in turn changes native LDL cholesterol to oxidized LDL. This leads to a chronic inflammatory response in the area around the lining of our arteries.

Step 3: Chronic Inflammatory Response

Chronic inflammation is the underlying cause of heart attacks, strokes, peripheral vascular disease, and aneurysms. These are altogether classified as cardiovascular disease (diseases that involve the arteries of our body). When inflammation of the arteries persists, the simple fatty streak I described begins to change. Not only does the inflammation attract more white cells (primarily monocytes), the monocytes then stuff themselves with more oxidized LDL cholesterol. This leads to a much thicker plaque, and the process of hardening of the arteries is now well under way.

This chronic inflammation also causes the muscle layer of the artery to thicken by a process called *proliferation*, the building up of more and thicker muscle cells. As a result, the artery begins to narrow. See Figure 3.

This entire process is a vicious cycle. Not only is there a buildup of plaque, but there is also a thickening of the artery. Normally, the layer of endothelium functions well by releasing an important product called *nitrous oxide*. During an inflammatory response, however, the appropriate release of nitrous oxide is blocked from the endothelium, causing the endothelium to function poorly. This in turn causes platelets to adhere to the plaque and the artery around the plaque to go into spasm.

Figure 3 — Clogged Artery

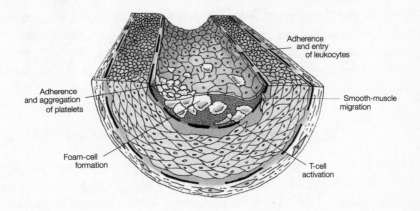

The foam-cells begin to accumulate, attracting in more monocytes, which eventually become foam-cells themselves. Smooth muscle begins to proliferate and also begins to migrate into this area and the lumen of the artery begins to narrow. The lining of the artery becomes more dysfunctional, which promotes further narrowing because of spasm of the artery and adherence of platelets.

Step 4: Plaque Rupture

The final event in about 50 percent of heart attacks is the rupture of one of these plaques and the clot that forms around a ruptured plaque. A situation such as this causes acute and abrupt total closure of this artery, which blocks the blood flow to that part of the heart. Potentially dangerous plaques are often small and may not even cause significant narrowing of the artery—making a diagnosis of heart disease difficult prior to the rupture of a plaque. (You can see now why this disease is so silent and unsuspected until the plaque ruptures and actually blocks the artery.) Oxidative stress may also cause the breakdown of these plaques, which eventually leads to their rupture.

Arteries can keep narrowing to the point that they become occluded (shut off). Have you ever had a friend or family member who had dye injected into his arteries to find out whether he had severe narrowing of one or all of his coronary arteries? These patients have usually had symptoms of chest pain or what doctors call *unstable angina*. In situations like these doctors either open vessels via angioplasty (ballooning of the artery) or bypass these blockages with surgery.

If you were to spend a day following a cardiologist or cardiovascular surgeon around the hospital, you would soon realize he has to spend the majority of his time "putting out fires." He typically treats patients who are at the end of the inflammatory process, with his entire focus on attempting heroically to save a life. Not much time is left to teach patients about the lifestyle changes necessary to slow down or even hopefully reverse this devastating disease and prevent the need for his services in the future.

True Prevention: What the Research Says

The good news is that antioxidants and their supporting nutrients can eliminate or at least significantly reduce *all* of the causes of inflammation in the arteries. Hundreds of clinical studies looking at heart disease report a significant health benefit with the use of nutritional supplements. Let's now look at each individual nutrient and see what its particular role is in slowing down or preventing this inflammatory reaction.

Vitamin E

Vitamin E is the most important antioxidant when it comes to hindering the process of hardening of the arteries. The main reason vitamin E provides such a powerful defense is the fact that it is fat-soluble, making it the most potent antioxidant within the cell wall. Vitamin E actually incorporates itself within the LDL cholesterol. The higher the vitamin E levels within the cell membrane of the native LDL cholesterol, the more resistant the LDL cholesterol is to becoming modified or oxidized. Wherever the native LDL cholesterol goes, the vitamin E travels right along with it.

It is important to understand that, as I mentioned earlier, LDL cholesterol does not become oxidized within the artery itself but only when it travels through the thin lining and into the subendothelial space. Researchers now believe that the high antioxidant content of the plasma or blood does not allow for this change to occur in the artery. In the subendothelial space the surrounding cells offer significantly less antioxidant protection. If the vitamin E content of the native LDL cholesterol is high, it is protected from becoming oxidized even if it passes into the subendothelial space.

Remember, the monocyte white cells pick up and drop off native LDL cholesterol so buildup doesn't occur. Keeping the native LDL cholesterol from being modified would prevent the entire inflammation process from the start.

Vitamin C

Recent studies show us that vitamin C is the best antioxidant within the plasma or fluid of the blood primarily because it is water-soluble. Vitamin C supplementation has been shown to preserve and protect the function of the endothelium.[7] Remember, endothelial dysfunction is at the core of this inflammatory process. Since maintaining the integrity of this thin lining of the artery is of utmost concern, numerous studies have appeared involving supplemental vitamin C to either prevent or decrease cardiovascular disease.[8]

Vitamin C has also been proven effective in protecting the LDL cholesterol from becoming oxidized within both the plasma and the subendothelial space.[9] Yet another benefit of vitamin C is that it has the ability to regenerate vitamin E and intracellular glutathione so they can be used again and again.

Glutathione

Glutathione is the most potent intracellular antioxidant and is present within every cell. Patients with known coronary artery disease have lower levels of glutathione within their cells than people whose arteries are healthy. Glutathione is a key antioxidant because it is contained in all the cells that surround the subendothelial space. When you take the nutrients needed for the cell to make more glutathione (selenium, vitamin B2, niacin, and N-acetyl-L-cysteine), you are improving the body's overall antioxidant defense system.

Bioflavanoids

Thousands of bioflavanoids exist within our fruits and vegetables. Here is a rule of thumb: the more varied the color of your fruits and vegetables, the greater variety of bioflavanoids you will get. These extremely potent antioxidants also have some antiallergen and anti-inflammatory properties. Red wine and grape juice have a product called *polyphenols,* for example, which have been shown to decrease the formation of oxidized LDL cholesterol. They also help protect the integrity of the endothelium.[10]

Grape-seed extract is believed to be the best bioflavanoid antioxidant in helping prevent chronic inflammatory disease.[11]

Nutritional Medicine: True Prevention

Research scientists are discovering that the root cause of heart disease is inflammation resulting from oxidative stress. Now clinicians (practicing physicians like me) need to take this information and make it practical and useful for you, the patient. But both physicians and researchers have a tendency to treat basic nutrients as drugs; that is, they test the body's response to just one nutrient at a time so they'll learn its exact potential.

For example, they will conduct a study with vitamin E, then a respective study will look at vitamin C, and then a separate study will examine the effects of beta-carotene. Occasionally a clinical trial does not show any significant health benefit and physicians and researchers hesitate in recommending that particular nutrient. This is what creates the controversy you see in the media and in the medical literature. Physicians want to know beyond any shadow of doubt that a particular nutrient will help before they will go on record to recommend any form of nutritional supplementation. But they are missing the all-important *synergistic effects* of nutritional medicine.

This refers to the ways antioxidants *work together*. To halt oxidative stress, the body needs enough antioxidants to handle all the free radicals, and the antioxidants need all of the supporting nutrients to do their job well. These ingredients work in synergy as they accomplish the ultimate goal of defeating oxidative stress.

I suggest that my patients provide all of the nutrients to the cell and tissues at optimal levels. I want to stop this inflammatory process from even getting started. Therefore, I recommend that they have the highest levels of vitamin E possible within the LDL cholesterol itself in order to protect it from becoming oxidized.

I have found my patients need to have optimal levels of vitamin C to protect the integrity of the endothelium, decrease the oxidation of the LDL cholesterol, and regenerate the vitamin E and glutathione. Beta-carotene, along with all the different types of carotene, is also necessary to help prevent or slow down this process.

I want to build up the glutathione levels within the cell by giving the body its precursors—selenium, vitamin B2, N-acetyl-L-cysteine, and niacin. In the next chapter, you will also learn the importance of folic acid and vitamins B6 and B12 in reducing the risk of cardiovascular disease.

Again, all of these nutrients work together either to eliminate or to decrease the inflammation in the arteries. The synergistic effect of supplementing all of these nutrients together is the key. That is why cellular nutrition is so critical to our health.

Turn the page and meet the new kid on the block . . . homocysteine.

SIX | Homocysteine: The New Kid on the Block

HAVE YOU EVER HEARD OF HOMOCYSTEINE? OR BETTER YET, HAS your doctor ever recommended a blood test to check your personal homocysteine level? Probably not. After reading this chapter I guarantee you will wonder why. Few people have ever heard of this substance, and fewer still realize that it poses just as great a threat as cholesterol when it comes to cardiovascular disease.

It is estimated that by itself, an elevated homocysteine level in the blood is responsible for approximately 15 percent of all the heart attacks and strokes in the world today—that means 225,000 heart attacks and 24,000 strokes each year in the U.S. In addition are the 9 million people who have cardiovascular disease as a direct result of elevated homocysteine levels.[1] Needless to say, I believe there is great value in learning more about this major killer, especially when you realize that you can correct it simply by taking B vitamin supplements.

What Is Homocysteine?

The history of homocysteine research is a fascinating one, beginning with the career of Dr. Kilmer McCully. A promising pathologist and researcher who graduated from Harvard Medical School in the mid-1960s, Dr. McCully enjoyed studies that involved the connection of biochemistry with disease. His reputation was strong, and he soon landed prestigious positions as an associate pathologist at Massachusetts General Hospital and as an assistant professor of pathology at Harvard Medical School.

Early in Dr. McCully's career, he became particularly interested in a disease called *homocystinuria*. This presented itself in children who had a genetic defect that kept them from breaking down an essential amino acid called *methionine*. These children showed a tremendous buildup of a by-product called *homocysteine*. McCully reviewed two separate cases involving young boys with this defect who died of heart attacks. This was quite amazing, since both of these boys were not even eight years old. When he examined the boys' pathology slides, he discovered that the damage to the arteries was eerily similar to that of an elderly man who had severe hardening of the arteries. This led Dr. McCully to wonder whether mild to moderate elevations of homocysteine that were present over a lifetime could be a cause of heart attacks and strokes in the average patient.[2]

As seen in the case of the two boys, homocysteine is an intermediate by-product that we produce when our bodies metabolize (break down) an essential amino acid called methionine. Methionine is found in large quantities in our meats, eggs, milk, cheese, white flour, canned foods, and highly processed foods. Our bodies need methionine to survive; however, as you can see from the list of foods that contain large quantities of this nutrient, we in the U.S. have plenty of it. Our bodies normally convert homocysteine into either cysteine or back to methionine again.

Cysteine and methionine are benign products and are not harmful in any way. But here is the catch: the enzymes needed to break down homocysteine into cysteine or back to methionine need folic acid, vitamin B12, and vitamin B6 to do their job. If we are deficient in these nutrients, the levels of homocysteine in the blood begin to rise.

So why haven't we heard of this before? We must turn back to Dr. Kilmer McCully.

Right Stuff–Wrong Era

McCully reported his homocysteine theory in several medical journals in the late sixties and early seventies and was initially welcomed with great enthusiasm. Dr. Benjamin Castle, the chief of his department, fully supported Dr. McCully and showcased his work to a prestigious panel of experts. But by the mid-seventies, the homocysteine theory had lost most of its momentum.

Dr. Castle retired, and the new chief of the department asked Dr. McCully to seek his own research funding or to leave. His lab was moved into the basement. McCully fought long and hard, but eventually time and money ran out:

in 1979 the new department chief informed Dr. McCully that Harvard was terminating him because his theory about homocysteine and heart disease had not yet been proven.[3]

Since McCully's positions at Harvard Medical School and Massachusetts General Hospital went hand in hand, he lost both jobs in January of 1979. A former classmate from Harvard who was then the director of the arteriosclerosis center at MIT labeled McCully's ideas "errant nonsense" and a "hoax being perpetrated on the public."[3] Soon the director of public affairs at Massachusetts General also asked Dr. McCully not to associate his homocysteine theories with the hospital or with Harvard.[4] McCully was shut down for good.

Dr. Kilmer McCully was certainly ahead of his time. But why the hostility toward a man who was simply trying to find the underlying cause of the number-one killer in today's world? What was the motive for such pessimism and verbal attacks? Could the heavily funded research on cholesterol at the time have been the reason?

At that time the cholesterol-heart attack theory was gaining tremendous momentum, and Kilmer McCully's hypothesis clearly challenged its future. Dr. Thomas James, cardiologist, president of the University of Texas Medical Branch, and the president of the American Heart Association in 1979 and 1980, said, "You couldn't get ideas funded that went in other directions than cholesterol. You were intentionally discouraged from pursuing alternative questions. I've never dealt with a subject in my life that elicited such an immediate hostile response."[5]

With all opposing theories silenced, the cholesterol theory went great guns. Drug companies began making their billions, and everyone was convinced that heart attacks and strokes were simply the result of too much cholesterol in the bloodstream. Wouldn't you say they did an excellent job in selling this to the medical community and to the general public?

Renewed Interest in Homocysteine

In 1990 Dr. Meir Stampfer revitalized interest in Dr. McCully's homocysteine theory. A professor of epidemiology and nutrition at the Harvard School of Public Health, Stampfer looked at the blood levels of homocysteine in fifteen thousand physicians who were involved in a health study. Dr. Stampfer reported that even *mildly elevated* levels were directly related to an increased risk of developing heart disease. Those men who had the highest levels of homocysteine experienced three times the risk of developing a heart attack when compared with those who had the lowest levels.[6] This was the first large study that showed the possibility of homocysteine as an independent risk factor for heart disease.

In February 1995 Dr. Jacob Selhub also reported in the *New England Journal of Medicine* that high plasma levels of homocysteine were directly related to an increased risk of carotid artery stenosis (the narrowing of the two main arteries supplying blood to the brain). In addition Selhub noted that most patients with high homocysteine levels also had low levels of folic acid and vitamins B12 and B6 in their bodies.[7]

Another large case-control study, The European Concerted Action Project, indicated that the higher the homocysteine level, the greater the risk of developing a heart attack.[8] What were once considered normal levels for homocysteine were suddenly becoming recognized as very dangerous levels.

Of even more concern to the researchers was the fact that when they found elevated levels of homocysteine in patients who also had one or more other major risk factors (hypertension, elevated cholesterol, or smoking), the risk of vascular disease increased *dramatically*. The results of these clinical trials provided evidence that the lower our homocysteine levels are, the better.

Suddenly researchers accepted as fact that homocysteine was indeed an independent risk factor for cardiovascular disease. Even the old-line supporters of the cholesterol camp, such as Claude L'enfant, director of the National Heart, Lung and Blood Institute, said, "Even if the risk of elevated homocysteine is not entirely proven, it is an extremely important area of research."[9] Today the medical evidence is beyond dispute: homocysteine can help cause coronary artery disease, stroke, and peripheral vascular disease.

Show Me the Money! The Economic Powers of Medicine

You can now appreciate why more than half the people who suffer heart attacks have normal cholesterol levels. Why did it take twenty-five years after Dr. McCully presented his hypothesis on homocysteine for the medical community to pay attention? Dr. Charles Hennekens, a professor at Harvard Medical School and chief of preventive medicine at Brigham and Women's Hospital, cites a parallel example. "For years now, we've known about these large benefits of aspirin in treating [patients] who have suffered an acute heart attack and survivors of heart attacks, and yet we have underutilization of it," he says. "At an FDA advisory committee meeting recently, I joked that if aspirin were half as effective, ten times as expensive and on prescription, maybe people would take it more seriously."[10]

Well, at least the pharmaceutical companies would take it more seriously, and they would definitely share those health benefits with the doctors. The situation here is similar. Like aspirin, at a cost of pennies a day vitamin B supplements can effectively lower the majority of elevated homocysteine levels. "It's inescapable that there's just not the commercial interest for supporting research in homocysteine," Dr. Stampfer says, "because nobody's going to make money on it."[11]

Take a look at the amount of money the medical community and the pharmaceutical industry have made by lowering cholesterol with synthetic drugs. Billions and billions of dollars roll in each and every year. Have you ever considered who educated you about the risk of high cholesterol? Who is taking out that full-page ad in USA Today to tell you the importance of lowering your cholesterol? Pharmaceutical companies. Why hasn't someone taken out a TV or newspaper ad to inform you about the importance of lowering your homocysteine? There is not nearly as much money to be made in the sale of vitamin B12, vitamin B6, and folic acid. Sad to say, we are caught in the ripple effects of the economics of medicine. Could this possibly have been the underlying reason that Dr. Kilmer McCully lost his research funds and his job at Harvard?

Dr. McCully takes his own follow-the-money approach, asking who stands the most to gain by not educating people about the dangers of homocysteine. "The most dramatic improvements in longevity over the last couple of hundred years have been through public health, not through medicine," he says. "But public health is notoriously unprofitable. People don't make a profit preventing disease. They make a profit through medicine—treating critical, advanced stages of disease."[12]

Is There a Healthy Level of Homocysteine?

Unlike cholesterol, which the body needs for the production of certain cell parts and hormones, homocysteine provides no health benefit. The higher the level of homocysteine, the greater the risk of cardiovascular disease. Conversely, the lower the level of homocysteine, the better. There is no threshold below which homocysteine becomes okay. You want your homocysteine level to be as low as possible.

Most labs will report the normal range of homocysteine levels between five and fifteen micromols/L (micromols per liter of blood). The medical literature finds that when this level rises much above seven micromols/L, however, an increased risk of developing cardiovascular disease becomes apparent. Most patients will want homocysteine levels below seven. If your level rises above twelve, you are in serious trouble.

Whenever the medical community discovers a new entity or risk factor, testing standards lag far behind. This happened with cholesterol and will happen with homocysteine. Therefore, do not be pacified by your physician, who might tell you that having a homocysteine level of ten or eleven falls well within the normal range and not to worry. You want to get your homocysteine level down to at least nine if you have no sign of cardiovascular disease; and below seven if you already have evidence of cardiovascular disease or have other risk factors of heart disease.

How Do I Lower My Homocysteine Level?

There are really two sides to this problem of high homocysteine levels. One is the amount of methionine in your diet that the body has to metabolize and break down. This requires that you become careful with the amount of meat and dairy products you are consuming. Isn't it interesting that these are the same foods that are high in saturated fat and cholesterol? Obviously, we need to replace these foods with more fruits and vegetables as well as vegetable protein. I realize that methionine is an essential amino acid; however, in the American diet, we will always get more than enough.

The other side of the coin is providing enough folic acid, vitamin B6, and vitamin B12 so that the enzyme systems needed to break down homocysteine can work effectively. It is interesting to note that all studies that have shown harmful aspects of elevated homocysteine have also shown depleted levels of B vitamins. I recommend that all of my patients take 1,000 mcg (micrograms) of folic acid, 50 to 150 mcg of vitamin B12, and 25 to 50 mg (milligrams) of vitamin B6.

Remember, the lower the homocysteine level, the better. I want to see everyone's level below seven if at all possible. When my patients have an initial homocysteine level above nine, I start them on supplemental B vitamins and recheck their blood level within six to eight weeks. With this B-vitamin regime, homocysteine levels tend to fall somewhere between 15 and 75 percent. But not all patients will respond adequately to just the B vitamins. This is an indication to me that these patients simply have an overall problem with methylation, the biochemical process used by the body to reduce homocysteine to benign or non-harmful products in the body.

Methylation Deficiency

Methylation deficiency is responsible not only for elevated homocysteine levels but is also one of the key underlying problems in some of our major chronic degenerative diseases, especially some cancers and Alzheimer's dementia. In fact as I am writing this chapter, a study has just reported that a new test has been discovered for determining who may be at higher risk of developing Alzheimer's dementia. I read the results of this study with great anticipation. Can you guess what the new test checks? Yes—the homocysteine blood level.[13] We have been doing this test in my office for the last several years because it points out the fact that elevated homocysteine levels are not only an indicator of vitamin B deficiency but also serve as an indicator for decreased levels of "methyl" donors in our body. Methyl donors are not only necessary to decrease homocysteine levels in the body, but they also produce important nutrients needed by the brain.

The least expensive methyl donor, which has an excellent effect on homocysteine levels, is called *betaine* or *trimethylglycine* (TMG). If the homocysteine level has not come down to the desired level, I add 1–5 g of TMG to the daily supplemental B vitamins.

Dr. Kilmer McCully: The Conclusion

A story was published on August 10, 1997 in the *New York Times Magazine* entitled "The Fall and Rise of Kilmer McCully." It detailed the end of his story and offered an interesting perspective to our concerns here:

> McCully reveals, briefly, the shadow of disappointment that must have loomed larger two decades ago. "Last October," he says, "the pathology department at Mass. General had a reunion and invited me, and I saw one of the people involved in my leaving the department. 'Well,' he said to me, 'it looks like you were right after all.' It's 20 years later. My career is almost over. There's really not much that can be done about 20 lost years, is there?"[14]

Worse, the political and economic forces that undid McCully back then may even be more intense today. Last April, the *New England Journal of Medicine* published an article titled "The Messenger Under Attack—Intimidation of Researchers by Special-Interest Groups," which detailed three cases of harassment by advocacy groups, physicians' associations, or academic consultants who often failed to disclose their close ties to drug companies. With more and more pressure groups weighing in on what research gets financed and promoted, the article said, "Such attacks may become more frequent and acrimonious."[15]

McCully knew the dangers of homocysteine. I'm sure he also knew that taking B vitamins in supplementation is not only inexpensive insurance against these dangers but safe as well. He was up against a political giant. But the truth is now clear. We are left to wonder why are doctors are still so reluctant to check their patients' homocysteine levels and why they are not recommending B vitamins to all of their patients. *What your doctor doesn't know may be killing you.* Especially when you consider the fact that homocysteine is an important, if not a greater, risk factor for heart disease than cholesterol.

The New Tests for Heart Disease

Ultrasensitive CRP

As the medical community begins to realize that coronary artery disease is decidedly an inflammatory and not a cholesterol disease, more clinical studies are appearing in the medical literature advising physicians of effective ways to evaluate patients. Several studies have looked at various products in the body that give us evidence of the amount of inflammation that is present in the arteries.

One such highly preferred blood test is the highly sensitive C-Reactive Protein (hs CRP). This test measures the arterial inflammation currently present. This test is actually a better predictor of who is going to develop heart disease than a cholesterol level is. Why shouldn't it be? In fact doing highly sensitive CRPs allows the physician to identify those patients who have normal cholesterol levels and may still be at increased risk of developing cardiovascular disease.

Homocysteine Blood Levels

Checking patients' fasting homocysteine blood levels is not only easy but also critical in determining whether they are problematic or not. Hopefully, as the test becomes more standardized between labs it will become more affordable. Presently, a serum homocysteine level test costs between $45 and $150.

Heart Calcification Scores

Most medical centers have now made modifications to their CT scanners so they can determine the amount of calcification, or plaque buildup, present in coronary arteries. This is a simple, noninvasive procedure, but its cost usually ranges between $250 and $600. I recommend this test for all patients with significant risk factors for or a strong family history of heart disease.

If the test does show calcifications, it gives a doctor some feel for how serious the problem is and how aggressively to treat the patient. Remember, more than 30 percent of the time the first sign of heart disease is sudden death. I have found this tool to be very helpful and motivating for my patients.

●　　●　　●

I challenge you to ask your personal physician to perform one or all of these tests on you. You may want to check with your insurance company first to make sure these tests are covered. Along with traditional chemistry profiles and cholesterol panels, these help determine which patients are at increased risk of developing cardiovascular disease. Obviously, it should be every doctor's focus to prevent or slow down this process in his patients so that they never have to end up in the surgeon's hands. Doesn't that appeal to you as well?

SEVEN | Cardiomyopathy: New Hope for a Cure

WAYNE IS A LIFETIME FRIEND. WE GREW UP TOGETHER IN A SMALL town along the Missouri River in South Dakota. His father was my baseball coach all the way through high school, and even though Wayne is younger than me, we always seemed to be competing neck and neck in sports. In fact when I was a senior, I set a local high school track record in the half-mile; Wayne broke it two years later. Wayne and I both went on to attend the University of South Dakota where we ran together on the USD track team. Following our years at the university, Wayne continued his athletic pursuits, was an aggressive cyclist, and still ran on occasion. I admired his continued drive to stay in peak physical condition.

Knowing his athleticism, then, I was quite concerned when my friend walked into my office one midsummer day. Wayne's color was poor, and he complained that his heart felt like it was going to jump right out of his chest. My former competitor looked tired and washed out as he informed me that he had come down with a severe flu about three months earlier and just never seemed to get over it. It seemed that anything he did completely wore him out. He was the manager of a restaurant and didn't know how he could continue working—it was that taxing to his body.

As I examined my friend, I noted right away that his heart was indeed beating rapidly and irregularly. Wayne's heart sounded like a washing machine. It was clear that he was in serious trouble, and I informed him that he needed to be admitted to the hospital.

Wayne went directly to the hospital, where one of our local cardiologists examined him. An x-ray revealed that Wayne's heart was significantly enlarged, so the doctor immediately ordered an echocardiogram (a sound-wave study of the heart). The results were shocking: Wayne's ejection fraction (a measure of how strong the heart is beating) was only 17 percent. A normal ejection fraction is between 50 to 70 percent. When an ejection fraction drops below 30 percent, the patient is a possible candidate for a heart transplant. Wayne's heart was huge, filled with blood clots, and in atrial fibrillation (beating irregularly). His situation was critical.

The cardiologist then performed a cardiac catheterization, in which he injected a special dye into Wayne's heart and coronary arteries. His arteries were fine, but his heart had definitely suffered trauma. The next test, a biopsy of the heart muscle, showed that as a result of suffering a viral infection of the heart, Wayne had developed cardiomyopathy (extreme weakness of the heart muscle). The infection had most likely occurred in the spring when Wayne contracted what he believed was the flu. He'd actually contracted a viral myocarditis, which caused severe damage to his heart.

The cardiologist prescribed the blood thinner Coumadin and placed Wayne on several other medications in an attempt to strengthen his heart. He was then able to leave the hospital, though he was very weak and could hardly move.

Follow-up studies of Wayne's heart a few weeks later showed that his ejection fraction had improved to 23 percent. The cardiologist wasn't very optimistic, though, and felt that this was probably the most Wayne's health would ever improve. His heart was still filled with blood clots, and he still was in atrial fibrillation.

The only other option the cardiologist had to offer was the possibility of sending Wayne to Abbott Northwestern in Minneapolis, where he could be put on a heart-transplant list.

You can imagine how difficult it was for me to discuss this with my patient, my friend. I also had to inform Wayne's parents, two people I had grown to love and admire, that their son's life was in serious jeopardy. To make matters more painful still, they had recently lost a younger son to lung cancer. It seemed like I was a messenger of hopelessness.

Wayne wanted to hold off going to Minneapolis and instead work with the local cardiologist and visit me on a regular basis. We placed him on a potent antioxidant and mineral supplement while he continued with his other medications. His blood clots finally cleared, and the cardiologist was able to convert Wayne's heart rhythm back to normal with electrical shock therapy.

About this same time my wife, Liz, and I were flying to the great Northwest when she showed me an article she was reading about a study on a natural nutrient, Coenzyme Q10. Liz handed me the article written by Dr. Peter Langsjoen, a cardiologist and biochemist practicing in Tyler, Texas. Dr. Langsjoen had been able to significantly improve the health of his cardiomyopathy patients by simply adding supplements of the nutrient called CoQ10 to their daily medications.[1]

As soon as I returned home, I thoroughly researched the medical literature about the use of CoQ10 and decided that it was safe to try with my friend. What did Wayne have to lose? I asked him into my office the next day and started him on a dosage of CoQ10 similar to what Dr. Langsjoen had been recommending.

Because Wayne was being so closely monitored by his cardiologist, I did not see him for three or four months, and when he did return to my office, he came to discuss the possibility of applying for total disability income. My hopes sank. *Total disability?* Wayne explained that because he had not worked for the past eight months, his friends and business acquaintances had strongly urged him to consider going on disability. When I asked how he was doing, however, he told me that he was feeling fine and was actually able to ride his bike an average of five miles a day. He was even able to run a little.

Grinning, I told Wayne that I would have difficulty recommending him for disability when his activity level had so dramatically improved. I suggested that we get another echocardiogram to see how his heart was doing. He agreed. I was astonished when I got the results. Wayne's ejection fraction was back into a normal range at 51 percent! The only explanation for his miraculous improvement was lots of prayer and the nutrient CoQ10.

The next week I ran into Wayne's cardiologist in the doctors' lounge, and I happily shared what had happened with our patient. But the cardiologist didn't reflect my enthusiasm. He simply did not believe me. In fact this doctor insisted that Wayne's echocardiogram be repeated on "his" machine.

Wayne was called to his cardiologist's office, but I didn't hear anything on the results for several weeks. When a letter finally did come, I learned that Wayne's ejection fraction on the cardiologist's machine was 58 percent. *Yes! That is even better,* I thought.

A week after I received the letter, I was grabbing a snack in the doctors' lounge when the cardiologist approached me. Our interaction was a bit different this time. Amazed at Wayne's improvement, the doctor was anxious to see some of the research studies on CoQ10. I told him I would send copies of the studies right over.

"Ray," he said, "you remind me of a doctor I used to listen to on the radio during my commute into work. He would talk about all these medical studies on nutrition and supplements. I was sure he was off his rocker. Slamming his topics became one of our favorite pastimes at the hospital. Man, we shredded him good."

The cardiologist continued, "The most critical doctor was Jim. In the doctors' lounge he would trash this radio guy up one side and down the next. This continued over the next few months until one day Jim's partner confronted him. 'Jim, if you feel this strongly about the subject, why do *you* take nutritional supplements?'

"'Well,' Jim replied, 'just in case I am wrong.'"

Wayne did not go on disability and is back to working full time. His first visit to my office occurred more than four years ago. My friend is now able to do all that he wants to physically and his follow-up echocardiograms continue to show that his ejection fraction is normal.

Let me assure you, though, that Wayne's heart has not been "cured." He still has cardiomyopathy. But with the addition of the nutrient CoQ10, Wayne's heart has its needed fuel source, which now allows his heart to compensate for its weakened state.

Diseases of the Heart Muscle

The heart is not a complicated organ. It is primarily a muscle whose main job is to pump blood throughout the body. In the last couple of chapters, we concentrated on the coronary arteries that supply blood to the heart. This chapter will now focus on the muscle of the heart itself.

Congestive heart failure and cardiomyopathy are diseases of the heart *muscle*.

An electrical system triggers this muscle to beat in a coordinated and efficient manner. The heart's valves then open and close, allowing the blood to flow efficiently through its four chambers. As the primary muscle with the responsibility of pumping life-giving blood to every organ in the body, the heart must continue beating consistently at all times and therefore has remarkably high energy requirements.

Congestive heart failure and cardiomyopathy have numerous causes: hypertension, repeated or severe heart attacks, viral infections, and infiltrative heart diseases like lupus or scleroderma, to name a few. In each case the disease weakens the strength of the heart muscle so that it is unable to handle the amount of blood it receives from the body. The heart tries to compensate for its weakened state by dilating and beating faster. But blood eventually backs up into the lungs, filling them with fluid. This is called *congestive heart failure*. The patient essentially begins to drown in his or her own fluid. Sometimes failure occurs primarily on the right side of the heart, which means the liver becomes congested and the patient's legs begin to swell.

When one's heart becomes severely weakened and dilated, as in Wayne's case, physicians call this cardiomyopathy. Cardiomyopathy is a very severe case of congestive heart failure. An uncommonly large, dilated heart is its hallmark.

What Is Coenzyme Q10?

Coenzyme Q10 (CoQ10), or ubiquinone, is a fat-soluble vitamin or vitamin-like substance that is also a potent antioxidant. Trace amounts of CoQ10 exist in a variety of foods, such as organ meats, beef, soy oil, sardines, mackerel, and peanuts. The body also has the ability to make CoQ10 from the amino acid tyrosine, but this is a complicated process that requires at least eight vitamins and several trace minerals to complete. A deficiency in any one of these nutrients can hinder the body's natural production of CoQ10.

Coenzymes as a group are cofactors essential for a large number of enzymatic reactions within the body. CoQ10 is the cofactor for at least three very important enzymes used within the mitochondria of the cell. Remember, the mitochondria are essentially the battery or furnace of the cell, where the energy of the cell is produced. Mitochondrial enzymes are needed for the production of the high-energy phosphate and adenosine triphosphate, upon which all cellular function depends.

You will recall that the mitochondria are where the oxidative process occurs. Not only does energy start here, but the dangerous by-products, free radicals, are also created. As a strong antioxidant, CoQ10 is extremely important in helping neutralize free radicals; however, its most important function in this situation is to help create energy.

CoQ10, which helps fuel human mitochondria, was first isolated from a beef heart mitochondria by Dr. Frederick Crane in 1957. In 1958, Dr. Karl Folkers and coworkers at Merck, Inc. determined the exact chemical structure of CoQ10 and began synthesizing it. The Japanese then perfected the technology in the mid-1970s and are now able to produce large amounts of pure CoQ10.[2]

CoQ10 Deficiency and Heart Failure

Not only have numerous investigators established the normal blood levels of CoQ10; they have identified what seems to be a direct correlation between the severity of heart failure and the correlating depletion of CoQ10. Significantly decreased amounts of CoQ10 have been noted in periodontal disease, cancer, heart disease, and diabetes. Deficient levels of CoQ10 have been most clearly established, however, in the blood levels of patients with congestive heart failure and cardiomyopathy.[3]

CoQ10 deficiency can be the result of several conditions: a poor diet, impairment of the body's ability to synthesize CoQ10, and/or the body's excessive utilization of CoQ10.

Investigators in the early 1980s began trials in which patients took CoQ10 supplements. Over the past twenty years, interest has continued to mount and numerous clinical studies have tested the results of CoQ10 in cardiomyopathy and congestive heart failure patients. No fewer than nine placebo-controlled clinical trials have taken place around the world. Eight international symposia have been held on the biomedical and clinical aspects of CoQ10, at which physicians and scientists from eighteen different countries presented more than three hundred papers.[4]

The largest of these international studies was the Italian Multi-Center Trial by Baggio and Associates, which involved 2,664 patients with heart failure. In this particular study nearly 80 percent of the patients improved when they started taking CoQ10, and 54 percent of these patients had major improvements in three major symptom categories.[5] Put simply, studies and real-life examples show that CoQ10 is an enormously helpful supplement in treating patients with life-threatening heart conditions. While it doesn't cure them, it certainly hinders the progress of the disease.

Treating Patients with Cardiomyopathy

Have you ever wondered what a heart transplant costs? Was your guess $250,000?

Were you aware that more than twenty thousand patients *under the age of sixty-five* are on the heart-transplant list? Thousands more patients over sixty-five also have cardiomyopathy, but they are not even eligible to be placed on the heart-transplant list because of their age. Although they may receive maximum medical treatment, most will remain totally disabled. Only one in ten patients who are eligible for a heart transplant will actually receive one; the other nine usually end up dying from their disease fairly soon. These numbers don't include the hundreds of thousands of patients who suffer from congestive heart failure.[6]

Drs. Folkers and Langsjoen reported a study in the medical literature in 1992 that I believe brings this dilemma to an obvious conclusion. They placed eleven exemplary transplant candidates on CoQ10. Three of the patients moved from the worst classification, Class IV, to the best classification, Class I, under the New York Heart Association guide (see box). Four patients improved from Class III–IV to Class II, and two others improved from Class III to Class I.[7]

The New York Heart Association classifications for functional capacity:

Class I: No limitations; ordinary physical activity does not cause undue fatigue, shortness of breath, or heart palpitations.

Class II: Slight limitation of physical activity; such patients are comfortable at rest. Ordinary physical activity results in fatigue, heart palpitations, shortness of breath, or angina.

Class III: Marked limitation of physical activity; although patients are comfortable at rest, less than ordinary activity will lead to the symptoms noted above.

Class IV: Inability to carry on any physical activity without discomfort; symptoms of congestive heart failure are present at rest. With any physical activity, increased discomfort and symptoms will occur.[8]

Against the backdrop of substantial clinical trials already reported in the medical literature, Folkers and Langsjoen showed undeniable proof of efficacy and safety of the use of CoQ10 in patients with end-stage heart failure who were awaiting transplantation.

Here is a prime example of a natural vitamin/antioxidant shown in several clinical trials to be effective and safe. This is nutritional medicine at its core. When the heart muscle is weakened, for whatever reason, it places an increased demand on the nutrients the heart cells need in order to create energy. Because of excessive utilization of these nutrients, the heart muscle eventually becomes depleted of CoQ10, which is the most important nutrient needed to create energy. When patients take this nutrient as a supplement, the weakened heart muscle is able to replenish its stores of CoQ10, generate more energy, and compensate for its weakened state.

Doctors should use CoQ10 in *support* of the traditional medical treatment, not in place of it. This is complementary medicine, *not* alternative medicine. Although in the studies many patients improved so much they were able to stop taking several of their medications, they were not cured of their underlying heart disease.

It is important to note that patients should continue taking supplemental CoQ10 over the long term. Clinical studies report that when patients discontinue using supplemental CoQ10, the needed fuel source becomes depleted again and heart function slowly decreases back to its previous poor level. On the other hand Dr. Langsjoen reported after a six-year follow-up study of patients that those who maintained their supplemental dosage maintained their heart function improvement.[9]

Why Don't Physicians Recommend CoQ10?

Here we have a life-threatening disease for which traditional medical therapy offers little hope for improvement. The cost of taking CoQ10 in supplementation is about a dollar (US) a day. Not considering the reduced costs of hospitalization, this is substantially less than the $250,000 heart transplant for which most of these patients are waiting! Furthermore, the use of CoQ10 has never shown any side effects or problems. In fact most of the studies show marked improvement within four months.[10] So why don't physicians recommend a trial of CoQ10 to their cardiomyopathy patients?

What doctors don't know may be killing you.

I have never heard a discussion of the use of CoQ10 at any medical meeting or with any cardiologist other than my interaction with Wayne's physician.

And I've never heard of a cardiologist placing any of my patients with congestive heart failure or cardiomyopathy on CoQ10. After reviewing these studies I too am amazed at the unwillingness of the medical profession to offer this option to their patients. Only 1 percent of the cardiologists in the U.S. recommend CoQ10 to their patients with heart failure or cardiomyopathy.[11] It is not as if they have a good alternative therapy in mind. The National Institute of Health has funded most of the studies involving CoQ10 in the United States. But unlike the plethora of synthetic drugs, CoQ10 is a natural product, and as such cannot be patented through the FDA.[12] Pharmaceutical companies are not going to spend the $350 million needed to get a natural product like CoQ10 approved by the FDA if there is no economic incentive.[13] It is also very costly for a company to promote the use of its medication to physicians. It is just not going to happen.

I'll tell you why physicians don't recommend CoQ10. Physicians are pharmaceutically trained. We know drugs, but we don't know much about natural products. As much as we hate to admit it, the pharmaceutical sales representatives who come to our offices daily control much of what we learn in regard to new treatments. And I have yet to see a pharmaceutical sales rep show me a study on CoQ10 and its effects on cardiomyopathy. There simply is no money in it.

Emma's Story

Emma is a delightful patient of mine in her early eighties. About four years ago, her cardiologist diagnosed her with cardiomyopathy. An ejection fraction of 20 percent severely limited Emma's life. Her cardiologist prescribed several medications, including Cardarone, which she took to control her irregular heart rhythm. However, this medicine made her very sick, and she was soon unable to eat. Not only did she lose a lot of weight, but the medication also destroyed her thyroid gland. Thyroid medication was started but, needless to say, Emma remained very ill. Her cardiologist did not give her much hope and, because of her age, she was definitely not a candidate for a heart transplant.

The traditional treatment Emma received only made her much worse.

In desperation she came to see me because she heard about how I was able to help others with similar problems. After evaluating my new patient, I could see she was having a significant reaction to the Cardarone. She wanted to quit taking the drug, and I agreed with her. I personally felt if she stayed on this medication she would live only another month or two. After easing her off Cardarone, I started my new patient on 300 mg of CoQ10.

To Emma's delight, her appetite and strength improved and her shortness of breath abated. Her activity level soon returned to normal. Four months later, her cardiologist repeated an echocardiogram and was pleased to see her ejection fraction had improved to 42 percent.

Emma has become more concerned about her arthritis than her heart. In fact she was able to have her left knee totally replaced—not bad for a lady who was not expected even to live!

It has been four years since Emma received her cardiomyopathy diagnosis, and she continues to live a healthy and happy life.

•   •   •

Physicians must become their patients' advocates. We need to learn and understand how natural products can help our patients. A basic principle here I cannot emphasize too much: when we support the natural function of the body and try to elevate its ability to perform at an optimal level, then and *only* then have we done everything possible to promote healing.

Taking supplements to accommodate this functioning is best described as complementary medicine. Patients with cardiomyopathy should continue taking their medication, but by adding a complete and balanced antioxidant and mineral tablet along with higher doses of CoQ10 (300 to 500 mg per day), we support the natural function of the failing heart, and the patient improves significantly.

EIGHT | Chemoprevention and Cancer

NOTHING IS MORE DIFFICULT FOR ME THAN HAVING TO TELL A patient he or she has cancer. Yet cancer is a diagnosis I must anticipate reporting as a routine part of my job. Doctors all over our nation have to share the same grim news with their patients: more than 1.3 million *new cases* will be diagnosed in the United States this year.[1]

Approximately 550,000 patients will die from cancer before the ball drops in New York City's Time's Square again. In spite of the $25 billion spent on cancer research in the past twenty years, deaths from cancer have actually *increased* over that same time period.[2] Major concern has arisen among researchers and clinicians alike—it's time to rethink our approach to cancer prevention and treatment.

But, you may ask, hasn't research made some great progress? Indeed. We have achieved some improvements, but those lie largely in the realm of being able to detect some cancers *sooner* through advances such as mammography for the detection of breast cancer and PSA tests for prostate cancer.

Is earlier detection all we can hope for? No. In this chapter we will discuss some of the most recent advances in cancer research and how you may be able to lower *your* risk of developing cancer.

Cancer and Its Causes

Doesn't it seem that just about anything we do or eat these days allegedly causes cancer? Excessive exposure to sunlight increases the risk of skin cancer. Asbestos workers have increased risk of developing an unusual form of lung cancer called *mesothelioma*. Smoking and secondary smoke are the main reasons lung cancer is the leading cause of cancer deaths. Radiation, charcoal steaks, too much fat in our diet, saccharin, and the many other chemicals found in herbicides and pesticides are what medical literature refers to as *carcinogens*, or those things that increase our risk of developing cancer.

Since the first report that chimney sweeps had an increased risk of scrotal cancer because of their exposure to soot,[3] we have become more and more afraid of our environment, and rightfully so. As I mentioned earlier, our bodies face exposure to far more chemicals than any previous generation's did. And what is the one common denominator all of these carcinogens have? You guessed it. They all increase oxidative stress. Here lies the key to understanding new strategies for fighting cancer.

Oxidative Stress as the Cause of Cancer

Many researchers have offered theories as to what is the underlying cause of cancer. Unfortunately, not one of these theories has been able to explain the completely diverse aspects of cancer and the development of the disease within the human body.

In response to this medical conundrum, Dr. Peter Kovacic authored a comprehensive review in *Current Medicinal Chemistry 2001*. There he stated, "Of the numerous theories that have been advanced, oxidative stress is the most comprehensive, and it has stood the test of time. It can rationalize and correlate most aspects associated with carcinogenesis (development of cancer)."[4]

Kovacic's research supports growing medical evidence that when excessive free radicals are allowed to exist near the nucleus of the cell, significant damage to the DNA of the cell can result. The DNA of the nucleus is especially vulnerable when a cell is dividing, during which time the DNA strand is literally unwound and stretched out. Researchers are now able to confirm not only that free radicals can damage the DNA nucleus of a cell, but also which strands of the DNA they damage most frequently.

When met with an onslaught of carcinogens, the body's MASH unit will be busy trying to repair the damaged DNA. But in times of heavy oxidative stress, free-radical damage overwhelms the repair system and can lead to mutation of the DNA. Free radicals can also wreak damage on the genetic structure of the DNA, which can then lead to abnormal growth of the cell. As these cells continue to replicate, this mutated DNA is carried to each newly developed cell.

When there is further oxidative stress to this mutated DNA of the cell, more damage occurs. The cell will then begin to grow out of control and take on a life of its own. It develops the ability to spread from one part of the body to another (metastasis), thus becoming a true cancer (Figure 1).

Figure 1

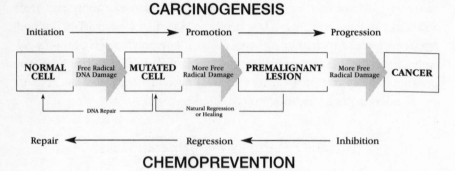

CARCINOGENESIS

A Multistage Process

Dr. Donald Malins, a biochemist from Seattle, reported a new method for identifying structural changes in the DNA of breast tissue. By using an instrument that bounces infrared radiation off the DNA and by analyzing the signals via a sophisticated computer, he is able to follow the structural damage to the DNA caused by free radicals.[5]

Researchers agree with Malins that the development of cancer is a multistage process that usually takes decades to develop. In adults cancer may take twenty or even thirty years to develop from the initial mutation of the DNA to its full-blown manifestation. In children this process may progress more quickly because of their more rapid cell turnover.[6]

Malins noted significant changes within the structure of the DNA as he followed it from normal breast tissue to metastatic breast cancer in all its developmental stages. Dr. Malins believed oxidative stress was the cause of this predictable damage to the DNA, which eventually led to the formation of breast cancer. He further argued that cancer was not so much the result of dysfunctional genes as it was the result of genetic damage that highly reactive free radicals caused.[7]

For the past twenty-five years, researchers have believed that abnormal genes are the driving force behind all cancers. But now researchers are beginning to believe instead that individuals with certain genes are simply more vulnerable to oxidative stress than others. This may explain the familial patterns of many types of cancer.[8]

A Decade Late and a Dollar Short

Physicians usually diagnose cancer in the last stages of its development. Unfortunately, by the time a cancer is advanced enough to cause symptoms or to show up on an x-ray, it has usually been developing for more than ten to twenty years. Doctors get out the big guns of aggressive surgery, chemotherapy, and radiation only to realize that most often they can do little to help the patient.

The last time I diagnosed lung cancer in one of my patients, his oncologist recommended chemotherapy, a procedure through which the physician claimed he could bring the lung cancer into remission about 40 percent of the time. My patient was somewhat encouraged by the statistics until he asked just exactly what was meant by "remission." The oncologist answered, "If the cancer is successfully brought into remission, your life can be extended by about three months." Needless to say, this was not what my patient had hoped to hear. This is the typical, tragic story for most people with cancer.

When my own mother was diagnosed with a high-grade brain tumor, the radiation therapist said there was about a 1 percent chance that therapy could prolong her life. Against my wishes, Mother went through the treatments. She died six months later after battling not only the cancer but also the treatments that left her weak and ill. An aggressive treatment may extend a life a few months to even a year or so longer, but the suffering our patients and loved ones must endure for the marginal benefits seems a cruelty to those whose lives are already so fragile.

We're presently losing the battle against cancer. Is there any doubt that this malignant disease must be attacked at *much* earlier stages in its development before the number of deaths will decrease? We do have hope, you know. Understanding the role of oxidative stress in the development of cancer offers us a host of new possibilities in prevention and treatment.

Prevention of Cancer = Chemoprevention

As we begin to understand the root cause of cancer, therapeutic options become available. Since cancer is a multistage process that takes years to develop, numerous opportunities arise to intervene in this process.

In the earliest stages of cancer, we see changes primarily within the DNA nucleus itself. The mutations that occur via the free-radical attack of the DNA pass to each subsequent cell as it replicates. Eventually, because of further free-radical damage to the cell, a precancerous tumor develops. This is the first practical level that we can evaluate clinically. The final stage is the development of a frank malignancy or cancer, which has the ability to spread from one part of the body to another.

Differing from attacking cancer with treatments in its final stages, chemoprevention focuses on preventing the cancer from developing in its earliest stages. Remember, balance is the key. If we have enough antioxidants available, oxidative stress does not occur and the DNA of the nucleus is safe from initial damage. Imagine again the metaphor of the fireplace. When a screen is in place, cinders cannot pop out onto the carpet.

Chemoprevention also aims to reverse the damage that has already occurred to the cell. As you learned in Chapter 4, the body has the amazing ability to heal itself (remember the MASH unit). Let us now carefully consider a strategy for fighting off cancer in three planned phases of chemoprevention, and the effects each has on the body.

Chemoprevention Phase I: Decreasing the Risk

The first strategy in the prevention of cancer may seem obvious: whenever possible, eliminate (or at least decrease) the exposure to carcinogens (chemicals that we know increase our risk of cancer). Though seemingly obvious, this phase is much easier said than done. Here are steps you should take immediately to decrease your risk of cancer:

1. *Stop Smoking!* Cigarette smoke is the most potent carcinogen to which many of us are exposed. Though nicotine is terribly addictive, we must struggle to rid the body of it and all the carcinogens contained in cigarette smoke. Smokers show a tremendous increase in the number of free radicals in their bodies.[9] And though to a lesser extent, secondary smoke is also an important factor in oxidative stress.[10]

2. *Reduce Your Exposure to Sunlight.* UVA and UVB ultraviolet light is a well-known carcinogen. I strongly recommend using sunscreen that protects against both. It's a discipline you can't live without. Parents, protect your children.

3. Eat a Low-Fat Diet. Excessive fat intake at meals is known to induce oxidative stress, especially when adequate amounts of antioxidants are missing in that meal. We must decrease saturated-fat intake, making certain we consume at least seven servings of fruits and vegetables and more than thirty-five grams of fiber each day. (I know you have heard all this before; but less than 9 percent of the population follows this advice!)[11]

4. Be Aware of Other Carcinogens. Whenever possible, choose to take action in decreasing your exposure to cancer-causing agents such as radiation, pesticides, herbicides, asbestos, charcoal, soot, and so on by purging them from your home environment.

A principle you will learn to appreciate is that if we reduce our exposure to *all* of these carcinogens, we will produce fewer free radicals for our body to fight. For example, it's difficult for me to recommend eating a healthy diet supplemented with nutritional medicine to a patient who is smoking two packs of cigarettes a day. I know the effect will be minimal at best; and unless he stops smoking, chances of decreasing the risk of cancer are definitely compromised.

Chemoprevention Phase II:
Maximize the Body's Antioxidant and Immune System

It is not possible to avoid exposure to all the carcinogens and chemicals in the environment. We must still live in this world. Hesitating with fear of "what might be out there" will only rob us of a full and abundant life. As you have already learned, the mere fact that we need oxygen to live puts us at a significant risk for oxidative stress. Therefore, the best strategy is not to hide out, but to maximize your own body's immune system and antioxidant defenses. And this begins by eating a healthy diet.

It seems logical that if *oxidative stress* is indeed the cause of cancer, *antioxidants* used to bring free radicals back into balance would lower the risk of cancer. This logic proves true. Cancer research specialist Dr. Gladys Block followed this precise logic while reviewing 172 epidemiological studies from around the world on diet and cancer. Dr. Block discovered a universal and consistent finding: those individuals who had the highest intake of fruits and vegetables (the main source of antioxidants) showed a significantly decreased risk of developing almost every kind of cancer. The risk of developing most cancers was *two to three times less* for those who had the highest intake of fruits and vegetables compared to those who had the lowest.[12]

The opposite also holds true. Dr. Bruce Ames, a leading cancer researcher, stated in an interview with the *Journal of the American Medical Association* that individuals who consume the least amounts of fruits and vegetables have twice the risk of cancer as those who consume more.[13]

Merely by consuming five to seven servings of fruits and vegetables daily, we can decrease the risk of almost every type of cancer by half.[14]

The absolute best defense your body has is a good diet. Nothing a doctor can prescribe will take the place of the diet your body needs to fuel and replenish itself. One of the principles you will hear me stress over and over is the fact that if you choose to use nutritional supplements, you must supplement a good diet, not a bad one. The first step toward building a strong immune system is to eat a high-fiber, low-fat diet largely made up of fruits and vegetables.

But we need more to practice chemoprevention. Medical research is beginning to demonstrate that taking antioxidants *in supplementation* to our diet is very important in chemoprevention. Studies show that supplementation of a good diet over a twenty-week period of time with vitamin C, vitamin E, and beta-carotene resulted in a significant decrease of the oxidative damage to the DNA of both smokers and nonsmokers. Vitamin E has also been shown to protect against exercise-induced DNA damage.[15]

Chemoprevention Phase III: Empowering the Body's Repair System

In Phase I and Phase II of chemoprevention, we were primarily concerned with decreasing the amount of oxidative stress the body has to handle and providing adequate antioxidants to prevent such stress to the DNA of the cell. In Phase III we will focus on the body's amazing repair system when coupled with adequate nutrients enabling the cell to repair significant damage that has already occurred.

Precancerous lesions or growths offer us a unique insight into the use of antioxidants in chemoprevention. It is difficult to follow these tumors within the body, but many studies have followed such tumors on the surface of the body. Such studies primarily look at leukoplakia, which is a precancerous tumor found inside the mouths of tobacco chewers, and cervical dysplasia, the precancerous tumor on the surface of the cervix.

We hope that by observing the use of various antioxidants on these tumors, we will gain insight into the possible effect on the already damaged DNA. Remember, cancer is a multistage process, and even precancerous tumors are in a relatively advanced stage. The next step in the multistage process is the development of a true cancer itself.

As you may imagine, great interest has piqued in the prevention and treatment of leukoplakia. Several studies have shown these tobacco chewers have low antioxidant levels. Consequently, those with the highest level of antioxidants also demonstrate the lowest risk of developing leukoplakia.

Dr. Harinder Garewal wrote a review article on the effect of antioxidants not only in the prevention of oral cancer but also the *reversal* of leukoplakia. This article is landmark to Phase III of chemoprevention. His findings provide hope that not only can antioxidants halt the process of developing cancer, they may actually empower the body's repair system to reverse cell damage.[16] I've briefly recapped in the box several of the clinical trials he studied.

Here is a list of studies that involve the use of nutritional supplements in patients with precancerous lesions:

1. A study in India used vitamin A and beta-carotene; researchers observed complete remission of the leukoplakia at a rate ten times greater than the placebo group.

2. A pilot study that used only beta-carotene showed a reversal of the leukoplakia back to normal cells in 71 percent of their patients.

3. In an ongoing study in the United States, patients received a combination of beta-carotene, vitamin C, and vitamin E; researchers witnessed a response rate of 60 percent. The abnormal precancerous cells reverted back to being normal cells.

4. In an ongoing multi-institutional U.S. trial, patients received only beta-carotene; they had a response rate of 56 percent.

5. A study done with male hamsters that had experimentally induced oral cancer considered using beta-carotene, vitamin E, glutathione, and vitamin C both in combination and alone. Significant improvement occurred in each group; however, the group receiving the combination had by far the best results. This was not merely an additional effect as more and more antioxidants were used but rather the results of a synergistic effect of the supplements working together.[17]

Cervical dysplasia is another precancerous tumor that occurs on the surface of the body. Several studies have shown that individuals with low levels of beta-carotene and vitamin C have significantly increased risk of cervical dysplasia. In fact women with the lowest levels of beta-carotene had two to three times more risk than women with the highest levels. Women who had an intake of less than thirty milligrams of vitamin C per day had a ten times greater risk of cervical dysplasia than women whose intake was higher. Other epidemiological studies have shown that dietary deficiencies in vitamin A, vitamin E, beta-carotene, and vitamin C increase the risk of cervical cancer. [18]

Beta-carotene supplementation actually has been shown to prevent cervical dysplasia from progressing to cervical cancer. In addition, some clinical trials have shown the role of vitamin C and beta-carotene in reversing or reducing the risk of cervical dysplasia altogether. [19]

Though medical science attempts to find the one "magic bullet" nutrient in each of these specific cancers, as a clinician, I try to determine *principles* that will be beneficial for my patient. After researching studies like the ones mentioned here, I have no doubt these antioxidant nutrients work together, in synergy. As I said in Chapter 5, this means we not only need an assortment of different antioxidants, but we also need the minerals (manganese, zinc, selenium, and copper) and the B vitamins that support their enzymatic functions.

I am awed by the incredible ability God has built into the body to not only protect itself against oxidative stress but to repair damage wrought on the DNA of the cell. Several ongoing clinical trials will further determine the roles of antioxidants in reversing this process of carcinogenesis. In the meantime, remember, leukoplakia and cervical dysplasia are at the very end of cancer's multistage process, and yet studies show how the body can repair itself when we provide it with optimal levels of a few select antioxidants.

What If I Already Have Cancer?

Granted, chemoprevention therapies really exist for individuals who have not yet developed full-blown cancer. And standard therapy for cancers doesn't always appear promising. These therapies involve surgery (when feasible), chemotherapy, and radiation for solid tumors such as cancers found in the lung, the breast, the colon, and so on. In spite of medical research efforts, these therapies seem to have reached a plateau.

The bad news continues. Despite evidence of increased cure rates in the treatment of Hodgkin's lymphoma, childhood leukemia, and testicular cancer, there is growing fear of the development of secondary cancers and complications that are the result of these treatments.[20]

The good news lies in the fact that medical research is beginning to support the idea of supplementation with a mixture of antioxidants and supporting nutrients. This mix can actually *enhance* traditional chemo- and radiation therapy while at the same time protecting normal cells from toxic effects.

Kymberly's Story

Kymberly was in her fourth year at Westmont College in Santa Barbara, California, working toward her degree in communication arts when she developed abdominal discomfort and bladder pressure. She went to the campus doctor, who diagnosed her as having a bladder infection and prescribed some antibiotics. But Kymberly's condition worsened. She experienced increasing abdominal pain, nausea, and vomiting.

While lying down, she was able to feel a mass in her lower abdomen. Obviously this frightened her terribly, and she went back to her doctor immediately. When he reexamined her, he could feel a mass the size of a grapefruit. He ran a blood test called a *CA 125*, which is a cancer marker for gynecological cancers and bowel cancers. Kymberly's marker was extremely high, and surgery was scheduled right away.

At age twenty-one, Kymberly had ovarian cancer. This being an unusual disease for such a young woman, the diagnosis caught her and her family totally off guard. After surgery the surgeon was quite optimistic that he had removed it all. He wanted to take every precaution, however, and requested that Kymberly see the oncologist. Her oncologist insisted that she go through some heavy chemotherapy, primarily because of her young age—she still had a lot of life ahead of her.

It was about this time that Kymberly consulted me. She wanted to know about nutritional supplementation as she was going through these treatments. She started an aggressive nutritional supplement program and scheduled her chemotherapy. Kymberly did not want to drop out of school, even though her doctors strongly recommended it. She was one student who was determined to give it her best shot, so she scheduled her chemotherapy treatments in Santa Barbara where she would continue to attend classes if it proved possible.

The young communications major did remarkably well through her treatments. She was able to carry a full load in college. Both Kymberly's oncologist and surgeon commented on not only how great she looked but also on how well she was tolerating her treatments. She did lose her hair, but she did not miss many classes. During her last treatment, the oncologist walked over to Kymberly and asked her directly, "What are you taking?"

Looking up, she replied, "What do you mean?"

He said, "I know you have to be taking something because all my other patients are over there vomiting, but you are here reading *Time* magazine."

When she told him about the nutritional supplements she'd been trying, he was impressed. Not only had she tolerated her treatments well, but she had *responded* so well to them.

Kymberly continues to thrive. It has been more than three years since she finished her chemotherapy. Her hair has come back beautifully, and she is enjoying life. Her CA 125 blood counts have remained normal, and she is now having them checked only twice a year. Kymberly has had no sign of recurrence of her cancer.

Why They Work

Oncologists and radiation therapists usually discourage the use of antioxidants in patients receiving treatments for their cancer. Why? Physicians are concerned with the possibility that antioxidant supplements will build up the antioxidant defense system of the cancer cells and result in making their treatments less effective, since their treatments primarily destroy cancer cells by creating oxidative stress. This is a reasonable concern. But the medical literature does not support their position.

Drs. Kedar Prasad and Arun Kumar and their colleagues at the University of Colorado Medical School Radiology Department reviewed more than seventy studies to address this concern. They titled their report, "High Doses of Multiple Antioxidant Vitamins: Essential Ingredients in Improving the Efficacy of Standard Cancer Therapy," which appeared in the *Journal of the American College of Nutrition*. There, Drs. Prasad and Kumar noted a few scattered studies that show a negative effect of using *one* nutrient in supplementation with certain chemotherapeutic treatments. When *high doses of multiple* antioxidants were used together, however, the therapies were enhanced.[21] Now why would this happen?

Antioxidants Help Destroy Cancer Cells

Clinical research is revealing that cancer cells take up antioxidants differently than do normal cells. Normal, healthy cells will take up only the amount of antioxidants and supporting nutrients they need. This is a very important scientific fact when it comes to the principles of cellular nutrition.

Cancer cells, on the other hand, continue to absorb antioxidants and supporting nutrients without knowing when to quit. This intake of excessive antioxidants actually makes the cancer cells more vulnerable to cell death. Antioxidants not only aid in the battle against cancerous cells, they improve the defense of healthy cells against the damaging effects of radiation and chemotherapy.

Antioxidants Help Good Cells

It is common knowledge that almost all of the harmful side effects of chemo- and radiation therapy to normal cells are the result of the increased oxidative stress these treatments create inside the body. What is not common knowledge, however, is that when a patient takes high doses of antioxidant supplements, he improves the defense system of normal cells since they take up these antioxidants normally. This creates a true win-win situation. Chemo- and radiation therapy can work at a peak while at the same time the terrible side-effects and damage that occurs to the healthy cells is significantly reduced.

Vitamin E protects against the damage caused by various chemotherapeutic agents to the lungs, liver, kidneys, heart, and skin. CoQ10 has been shown to protect against the long-term damage to the heart that the drug Adriamycin causes. Beta-carotene and vitamin A reduce the adverse effects of radiation and some chemotherapeutic agents. All of these antioxidants have been shown to help protect against the DNA damage to normal cells that cancer treatments cause.

Michelle's Story

Michelle was a beautiful, vibrant four-year-old. Her world was filled with love and lots of laughter. It appeared that nothing could penetrate the safe haven of her family. But Michelle's carefree life changed. Doctors discovered the discomfort she was experiencing in her back and abdomen came from an aggressive cancer called a *neuroblastoma*. The family was devastated.

Michelle underwent exploratory surgery shortly after the diagnosis. When the surgeon emerged from the operating room, the family could see from his face that the news was not good. He informed them that Michelle's tumor had spread, stretching clear up to her diaphragm, and had wrapped around the bowel and the large vein in her abdomen. There was no way he could remove it.

Before Michelle even recovered from her exploratory surgery, her oncology team started her on aggressive chemotherapy but still was not optimistic about Michelle's chances for long-term survival. This was when Michelle's mother consulted me. She wanted to do everything possible to protect her daughter from the potential side effects of the treatments the doctors recommended.

We started Michelle on an aggressive nutritional supplement program in spite of her doctor's objections. Michelle was a trooper and took her supplements faithfully. Her treatments began, and she struggled through them. She did become fairly sick even though she was taking the supplements. Because the treatments were exceptionally strong, there was serious concern that she could actually survive them. But brave little Michelle made it through, and the tumor shrunk significantly.

Michelle's response so encouraged her doctors that they wanted to take her back into surgery to see if they could remove the tumor. This time the surgeon emerged from the OR with a smile on his face. He said they felt they were able to get all of the tumor. The oncologist informed Michelle's parents that her response to the chemo could not have been better.

But Michelle's journey was not over. The doctors still wanted her to go through a bone marrow transplant to ensure that any microscopic spread of the cancer was removed. The family faced another tough decision. They carefully considered all the information they could gather, and then based on that information, Michelle's father told the oncologist that they would consent to the bone marrow transplant. The physician could proceed on one condition only: Michelle's parents insisted that she be on nutritional supplements during the bone marrow transplant.

At first the oncologist refused. She believed the nutritional supplements would block the effectiveness of her treatments. When Michelle's father asked the oncologist if she had any studies in the medical literature that supported her concerns, the oncologist replied, "No, but it is a theoretical concern."

Then Michelle's father, who was also an ER physician, revealed that she had been taking supplements all during her previous treatment. She had not only survived the treatments but experienced an exceptional response. Michele's father made it clear that he and his wife insisted that she stay on the supplements while going through the bone marrow transplant.

The oncologist agreed to have the oncology pharmacologist investigate the supplements Michelle was taking to be sure there would be no conflict with the drugs. After extensive research by the pharmacologist, all agreed that Michelle could receive supplements during the bone marrow transplant after all. The procedure was rough, but she survived, and she did recover. In fact the oncologist told the parents that she had never seen any child recover more quickly from such a procedure. Their tough stand had been well worth the effort.

Michelle and her mother prayed many times through those difficult months that when she turned five, she would be able to start kindergarten with her friends. And Michelle was strong enough to make that first day of kindergarten. It has been more than three years since she was first diagnosed with the cancer. At age seven Michelle is busy riding bikes, jumping rope, and keeping up with fashion and her girlfriends.

* * *

Nutritional science offers us the greatest hope in our fight against cancer and several other degenerative diseases. They not only help prevent cancer but may actually enhance the traditional chemo- and radiation therapy. How can the process of building up the body's natural defense be bad? Shouldn't physicians want their patients to be as healthy as possible, since cancer treatments are going to put patients under the greatest stress they have had to endure in their lives?

Natural antioxidants and their supporting nutrients are the ideal chemopreventive agents for many reasons. They

- limit and even prevent the free-radical damage to the DNA nucleus of the cell.

- provide the proper nutrients needed for the body to repair any damage that has been done already.

- are safe and may be taken over a lifetime. (Pharmaceutical drugs do not share this advantage. Tamoxifen, which has been shown to decrease the risk of breast cancer, has very serious side effects.)

- are relatively inexpensive. (The nutrients I recommend for prevention cost between $1.00 and $1.50 (US) per day.)

- provide the best defense against further advancement of cancer.

- protect the body against oxidative stress that chemotherapy and radiation create.

- embellish the cancer-fighting ability of chemotherapy and radiation.

- inhibit the replication and growth of the cancer.

- have been shown to cause tumor regression in some instances.[22]

We cannot deny that the effectiveness of traditional cancer treatments has reached a plateau. Oncologists and radiation therapists must become more open-minded about antioxidant use in their patients. As researchers seriously consider the use of multiple antioxidants at optimal levels, cancer prevention and treatment may well be revolutionized. In the meantime the research that is presently available supports the use of antioxidants in all stages of chemo-prevention and cancer therapy.

NINE | Oxidative Stress and Your Eyes

NOTHING COULD SLOW MAVIS DOWN. AFTER LOSING HER HUSBAND many a year ago, she had grown tough and independent. She loved to travel and ventured out on her own without a trace of hesitation. Mavis knew what living was all about.

No, nothing could slow Mavis Ehresman down . . . except the dark fear of approaching blindness. Back in 1983, Mavis, who loved to watch lightning storms split the night sky, who could distinguish subtle differences in the seemingly endless landscape of wide-open prairies, noticed she was having a difficult time seeing. When her sight didn't get any better, she decided it was time to make a trip downtown to visit the local eye doctor.

He diagnosed her that day with macular degeneration. And everything seemed to move in triple slow motion as she made her way back to her car.

Though Mavis was not familiar with this particular problem, she knew she must use the eyesight she had left—and time was running short. She brought herself up to speed by reading everything she could about her disease. If there *was* a solution to be found, Mavis would find it.

But what she read wasn't good. The books said doctors could do nothing for her but watch her vision deteriorate. And that is exactly what happened.

Over the next fourteen years, Mavis's eyesight continued to decline. At first she had to give up night driving. Then she found that driving in the winter became impossible too because the gray skies would blend with the road. Winters last a long time in South Dakota.

The old Chevy now remained parked in the driveway. But the same gritty determination that drove Mavis through many a blizzard drove her to find solutions. On an April day in 1997, my phone rang, and Mavis spoke up. She'd called the right place. After sharing with the South Dakota woman everything in this chapter on macular degeneration, I explained the recommended doses of nutritional supplements. Mavis started taking a potent antioxidant and mineral tablet along with high doses of grape-seed extract.

Within a couple of months, Mavis's vision began to improve. Her eyesight became clear, and even her night vision got better. She was thrilled the next time she visited the local eye doctor because he confirmed the good news. In fact her vision that day was at the same level as it had been back in 1991—six years prior!

The old car didn't sit in the driveway anymore. Mavis had places to go— things to see. Winter and nighttime driving were still a concern, but the old gripping fear of losing her vision didn't slow Mavis down anymore. This hard-charging woman who knew how to live looked again in awe at the huge night skies and wide-open prairies until the Lord took her home in the fall of 2001.

The Problems Eyes Have

The role of oxidative stress as the cause of degenerative changes in the eyes has generated significant interest in the use of antioxidant vitamins and minerals as a means of preventing or even treating age-related eye diseases. No fewer than six large, multicentered clinical trials are presently ongoing to study carefully the use of various nutritional supplements in the following diseases.[1]

Cataracts

Cataract surgery is the most common surgical procedure for patients more than sixty years of age. Its economic impact on the U.S. health-care system is tremendous. In the United States eye surgeons perform 1.3 million cataract surgeries each year at a combined cost of more than *$3.5 billion*. It has been estimated that a ten-year delay in the development of cataracts in the U.S. population would eliminate the need for nearly half of these surgeries.[2]

The lens of the eye collects and focuses light on the retina. In order to perform its job properly, it must remain clear throughout our lifetime. As we age, various components of the lens may be damaged and opacities may occur, leading to age-related cataracts.

Medical researchers believe it is essential to determine if supplying adequate levels of antioxidant nutrients to the eyes *early in life* will preserve lens function, protecting them from cataract formation. Basic research studies support the theory that free radicals are once again the culprit; they arise from ultraviolet sunray damage and form cataracts.[3]

The natural antioxidants the body makes (glutathione peroxidase, catalase, and superoxide dismutase) form the eye's primary defense system. But researchers have realized that the *natural* antioxidant defense system is not adequate in fully protecting the eye. In fact several clinical trials have considered the possibility that increased dietary and supplemental antioxidants may be protective against oxidative damage to the lens.[4]

Antioxidants found in the fluid around the lens of the eye are critical in protecting the lens itself. Thus, cataract development takes place at a much faster rate if this fluid around the lens contains low levels of additional antioxidants. The most important antioxidant in this fluid is vitamin C. Vitamin C is water-soluble and is found in high concentrations around the lens. Other antioxidants found in this fluid are vitamin E, alpha-lipoic acid, and beta-carotene.

Several epidemiological studies have demonstrated the association between the levels of vitamin C, vitamin E, and beta-carotene and the risk of developing cataracts. In Finland a case-controlled study showed individuals who had the lowest levels of vitamin E and beta-carotene had a four- to five-fold increased risk of needing cataract surgery.[5] Another study showed that those individuals who consumed supplemental vitamins had at least a 50 percent decreased risk of developing cataracts.[6]

Good medical evidence exists showing that the natural antioxidant protection of young lenses decreases significantly with age. Several different clinical studies provide evidence that when people use various antioxidant supplements, this protects the aging eye. Researchers have found the higher the level of vitamin C found in the aqueous fluid around the eye, the greater the protection against cataract formation.[7] Because of its synergistic effect, alpha-lipoic acid has been shown to embellish the work of all these antioxidants in protecting the lens of the eye. Recent clinical studies also reveal that both alpha-lipoic acid and vitamin C have the ability to regenerate the intracellular glutathione so it can be used again and again.[8]

I only hope that over the next few years all physicians will recommend antioxidants as a way to protect against cataracts. As clinical trials begin to report their findings, we'll know more about specific antioxidants and the supplemental levels of these antioxidants. But I believe sufficient evidence exists *now* to warrant encouraging patients to consume antioxidant supplements as a relatively inexpensive way to decrease this high incidence of cataract formation.

Macular Degeneration

In the United States, age-related macular degeneration (ARMD) is the leading cause of blindness in people more than sixty years old.[9] For those who are not familiar with this disease, it is a decay of a critical part of the retina called the *macula*. This is where the greatest concentration of photoreceptors is located and is the area responsible for central vision. When this area of the eye begins to decline, we essentially lose central vision, our most important aspect of sight. If an individual with ARMD were to look right at you, he would not be able to see your face but could see things around you. In other words peripheral vision remains intact.

Macular degeneration presents itself in two different forms: wet and dry. Ninety percent of cases involve the dry form, in which central vision gradually reduces and may progress to the wet form about 10 percent of the time.[10] No proven treatment for the dry form of macular degeneration currently exists.

The wet form causes a more rapid reduction in central vision, the development of new vessels, and possible vessel leakage. The wet form of macular degeneration is potentially treatable via laser photocoagulation. This treatment attempts to slow the new vessel production, which causes swelling (edema) and leakage or bleeding into the retina, and to stop the bleeding this leakage may cause. Blindness usually still follows rather quickly, however.

Prevent Blindness America estimates that 14 million Americans have evidence of ARMD. The Beaver Dam Eye Study reports that 30 percent of the people in the U.S. over the age of seventy-five have ARMD and 23 percent of the remainder will develop ARMD within five years.

Mechanism of Injury to the Retina

In recent years several researchers have made interesting proposals as to the actual cause of age-related macular degeneration (ARMD). These theories suggest that light that enters the eye and is focused on the macula of the retina causes significant free-radical production in the outer aspect of these photoreceptors. Again, if antioxidants are not available to readily neutralize these free radicals, the free radicals can cause damage to the

---

photoreceptors. This form of oxidative stress has also been shown to create damage to the high concentration of polyunsaturated fats (PUFAs) in the outer retina and photoreceptors.

Much like the oxidation damage to the LDL cholesterol, the oxidized and damaged PUFAs cause the formation of lipofuscin—a group of lipid/protein products that are collected within the retinal pigment epithelium. Lipofuscin creates even more oxidative damage to the retina, and researchers believe it is actually the cause of damage to and destruction of these sensitive photoreceptors.

These toxic substances can accumulate in the pigment epithelium cells and are eventually excreted in the form of drusen. Drusen formation is one of the first indications to an ophthalmologist that a patient is developing ARMD. As these drusens accumulate between the pigment cells and their blood supply, they block the exchange of nutrients and the photoreceptor cells can no longer function, causing an area of blindness.

Damage to the Photoreceptors

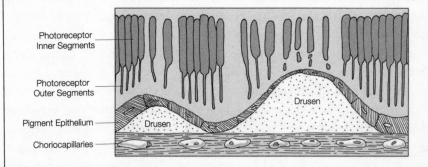

The development of drusens separates the photoreceptors of the eye from its blood supply and causes an area of blindness.

The Generation of Free Radicals in the Retina

As I stated, when the retinal pigment and photoreceptors absorb light, the process forms free radicals. High-energy ultraviolet light and visible blue light are especially capable of producing enemy free radicals in the retina of the eye. As you may guess, patients exposed to this high-energy light over an extended period of time have a significantly greater risk of developing

ARMD. Studies suggest that as we get older, the antioxidant defense systems that protect us against the free radicals caused by high-energy light waves declines significantly.[11] This obviously upsets the balance our body creates between antioxidants and free radicals and leads to increased damage to the retina of the eye.

Several studies have shown that people with macular degeneration had low levels of zinc, selenium, vitamin C, carotenoids, and vitamin E when compared to people who did not have macular degeneration.[12] Clinical studies examined the effects of supplementing individual nutrients to see if they could improve or slow down the development of ARMD. Following is a condensed compilation of the results.

Carotenoids

"Now, Ray, eat your carrots. They're good for your eyes." I can still hear my mother urging me to eat my creamed carrots before I could get down from the table to play.

Did your parents ever tell you to eat carrots too? Doctors believed then that the beta-carotene found in carrots was necessary for good eyesight and night vision. This is true to a degree, but beta-carotene is only one of a dozen important carotenoids found in the body. It is actually more important to eat corn, leafy green vegetables, and collard greens because they contain high levels of carotenoids called *lutein* and *zeaxanthine*.

Because lutein and zeaxanthine are yellow, they efficiently absorb the blue light portion of visible light. Blue light is the major high-energy light that can damage the lens and the retina of the eye. When these two nutrients are present in the lens and macula, our eyes absorb blue light and minimize oxidative stress. They essentially act like internal sunglasses. They screen out the harmful, high-energy light and decrease the number of free radicals that the photoreceptor cells produce. These nutrients are also very potent antioxidants and as such are able to help neutralize any free radicals that occur in this area of the eye.

Studies Show Lutein Helps Protect the Eye

Patients who took lutein and zeaxanthine in supplementation were not only able to raise their blood levels of these nutrients but also significantly increased the levels within the eye. Macular pigment, which protects the

---

retina from being damaged, increased 20–40 percent in these studies, while blue light transmitted to the macular photoreceptors and macular pigment decreased nearly 40 percent.[13]

The *Journal of the American Medical Association* reported in its November 9, 1994, issue that patients who had the highest intake of the two yellow nutrients, lutein and zeaxanthine, from their diet had a 43-percent decreased risk of developing ARMD over those who had the lowest intake. Interestingly, these same benefits were not apparent with patients who had high levels of beta-carotene. Lutein and zeaxanthine are the only carotenoids that are specifically deposited within the macula of the eye.[14] Though beta-carotene found in creamed carrots is healthy for us to eat, it will not provide a decreased risk of ARMD. Perhaps what Mom really meant was, "Eat your carots"—as in carotenoids.

Vitamin C

People with low levels of vitamin C have an increased risk of developing ARMD. Vitamin C is highly concentrated in the fluid within the eye (aqueous humor) and is a very important antioxidant for the retina. Studies indicate that supplementation with vitamin C can slow down the progression of ARMD. Vitamin C also has the ability to regenerate both vitamin E and the potent intracellular antioxidant glutathione.[15]

Vitamin E

ARMD patients have low levels of vitamin E in the area of macula, where high-energy light produces excessive free radicals that damage the photoreceptors. Even though vitamin E is not the most important antioxidant within the eye, it is still a critical player. When a patient takes vitamin E in supplementation, he may provide protection against the development of ARMD.[16]

Coenzyme Q10

By now you are familiar with CoQ10 from the discussion on cardiomyopathy in Chapter 7. CoQ10 is a potent antioxidant that is fat-soluble. This nutrient has been found to be a great protector of fats throughout the body. The retina of the eye, which is made up in large part by fat, is no exception.

Patients with ARMD show significantly depleted amounts of CoQ10. Those patients with normal levels of CoQ10 have greater capacity to resist oxidative damage that excessive free radicals cause.[17] CoQ10 is new in the study of ARMD, and its effects appear promising.

Glutathione

Glutathione is a very potent antioxidant found within every cell in the body. It is especially critical within the lens of the eye as well as the pigment and photoreceptor cells of the retina. Clinical studies have shown that as we age, the level of glutathione declines. This fact is imperative to consider in relation to the increase of diseases in the eye as we age. Several studies have looked at trying to increase the level of this crucial antioxidant within the lens and retina of the eye.

Among researchers, it is a well-known fact that our body absorbs oral glutathione poorly; raising cells levels of glutathione via this method are next to impossible.[18] The best way to increase intracellular glutathione levels is to provide nutrients that the body needs to manufacture its own glutathione. Remember, glutathione peroxidase is one of the natural antioxidant defense systems that the body creates. The nutrients needed for the body to make its own most effective, natural defense are selenium, vitamin B6, N-acetyl-L-cysteine, and niacin.

As you learn more about cellular nutrition, you will begin to realize the importance of providing all of these precursor nutrients to the cell. In this case alpha-lipoic acid and vitamin C are also critical because they both have the ability to regenerate glutathione. Since it is difficult to increase the levels of glutathione within the cell, these nutrients should also be present in supplementation so that the glutathione can be used again and again.

Researchers have demonstrated that when the photoreceptor and retinal pigmented cells have optimal levels of antioxidants present, they are much better able to protect these cells from oxidative damage. The lens of the eye is also better protected against oxidative damage when glutathione levels are higher.[19]

Zinc and Selenium

Zinc and selenium are important minerals our antioxidant system needs. Zinc is critical for the function of our catalase antioxidant defense system and selenium is necessary to the glutathione peroxidase system. Both of these antioxidant defense systems are essential in the battle against free radicals produced in the eye. If these two minerals are not available in adequate amounts, the two defense systems simply cannot perform at their optimal level. Several studies now show that when these minerals are supplemented, especially zinc, ARMD can actually be stabilized and improved.[20]

Faye's Story

One of my longtime patients accompanied her husband for a checkup. During that visit, Faye told me that she had just been diagnosed with macular degeneration.

While traveling to Texas to see family, she noticed that she just could not see anything clearly. She kept wiping off her glasses and putting them back on only to find that she still could not see well. She decided at that time she needed to get her glasses prescription changed. When she got back home she went to see her local eye doctor, who couldn't find anything wrong.

But Faye's sight got worse. When she went to church, she couldn't make out the faces of the people in the choir. Worried, she made an appointment with a local ophthalmologist who specialized in retinal diseases. He examined her and right away diagnosed macular degeneration. Faye had already lost quite a bit of vision in her left eye, and the physician informed her that she had the wet kind of macular degeneration. He would need to follow it closely in case she would need any laser treatment.

I explained to Faye the research I had done with macular degeneration and how several of my patients were able to actually get visual improvement by taking nutritional supplements. Obviously, she wanted to try them so I started her on the supplement program outlined in Chapter 17.

Within two months Faye shared with me that she had significant improvement in her vision and that it was even getting close to being normal. She was now able to see every face in the choir.

This story took place five years ago, and Faye continues with the nutritional supplements. Her vision has basically remained stable. Faye continues to make appointments with her ophthalmologist every few months but still has not needed any laser surgery. Her doctor tells her that her eyes look beautiful.

Protecting Your Eyes Against Cataracts and Age-Related Macular Degeneration

I have shared a lot of technical information with you. But I have done this so that you will have the medical evidence you need to know to make solid decisions about nutritional supplements and avoiding eye disease. These recommendations also apply to those who already have cataracts or macular degeneration and desire to slow down those processes. But I anticipate that you may be wondering, *How do I make all this practical?*

In my clinical practice I am markedly aggressive with my macular degeneration patients because I want to see if we can actually reverse some of the damage that oxidative stress has caused. I have personally been involved with more than a dozen patients whose ophthalmologists have documented visual improvement after following these recommendations.

First of all, it is critical for all of us to protect our eyes from the damaging high-energy sunrays that are the underlying cause of oxidative stress in our eyes. In a healthy young adult, the cornea and lens of the eye, which protect the retina, absorb most of this UV light. But the cornea and lens do not block or absorb the high-energy visible blue light. As we age, the lens of the eye allows more and more ultraviolet light through and no longer protects the retina from this threat.

When it comes to protecting your eyes, the enemy is sunlight. It is very important that we decrease the amount of oxidative stress our body needs to handle. Purchasing high-quality sunglasses that block all UV light and the visible blue light is a great investment. This means that you do not have to neutralize as many free radicals.

Clinical studies concerning the eyes indicate that when the antioxidant defense system becomes overwhelmed, everything breaks down and oxidative stress occurs. We all need to become more conscientious about shading our eyes and face from direct sunlight. People who work outdoors, or those who are involved in sports and activities where they are exposed to intense sunlight, should especially wear protective eyewear at *all times* while outside.

The other half of the equation is again to build up our body's natural antioxidant defense system. Several studies have shown that by taking nutritional supplements we are able to do this. In one particular study 192 patients with macular degeneration took antioxidants and 61 control patients didn't. After six months 87.5 percent of the supplemented patients had visual acuity equal to or better than at the beginning of the study. Only 59 percent of the untreated group had visual acuity equal to or better than at the beginning of the study.[21]

Again, I outline what antioxidants to take for this in Chapter 17.

•   •   •

Two years ago, one of the ophthalmologists in town stopped me in a restaurant parking lot. He asked, "What is this nutritional stuff you recommend to your patients with macular degeneration? I just saw a lady in my office this morning whose vision improved from 20:100 to 20:40 in both eyes. I have never seen this before in patients with macular degeneration."

I explained briefly the concepts presented in this chapter.

Reaching for his sunglasses, the ophthalmologist opened his car door. With a wink and a smile he said, "You can help all the macular degeneration patients you want, but don't help those patients with cataracts. We can always operate to help them."

I knew he was only joking, and I appreciated his genuine interest in nutritional supplements. Since there is little doubt that the underlying cause of cataracts and macular degeneration is oxidative stress, I believe that we must be nothing short of aggressive in our supplementation program. After all, there really is no other effective treatment for ARMD and many patients could avoid needing cataract surgery altogether. Can such a simple solution offer any better results than that?

TEN | Autoimmune Diseases

BEING THE YOUNGEST OF SIX CHILDREN, MARK HAD TO BE TOUGH just to keep up with the others. He was a healthy little guy who loved anything that had to do with playing ball and a good bit of competition. He was involved in several sports, but soccer was his all-time favorite.

One day when Mark was twelve years old, he was aggressively running the ball in soccer practice when he started cramping up. Soon he was doubled over with severe stomach pains. The cramps continued to mount over the next few days with both diarrhea and vomiting. When Mark didn't respond to any over-the-counter medications, his parents finally took him to the emergency room where he was diagnosed with appendicitis. After a brief surgery and recovery, Mark was released from the hospital.

He wasn't home for long. He returned to the hospital within twenty-four hours due to increasing abdominal pain, bloody diarrhea, and vomiting. Mark was now much sicker than he was before the operation.

The young boy was readmitted to the hospital; however, the local doctors were puzzled. They referred Mark to the pediatric gastroenterology department at Loma Linda University Medical Center; there doctors placed him immediately in the pediatric intensive care unit. They performed a colonoscopy the next day and took several biopsies of his small bowel and colon.

What his parents saw during the procedure on the video display made them stare in disbelief. Later they described to me how the entire lining of Mark's bowel looked like a cobblestone street. The Loma Linda physicians diagnosed Mark as having an autoimmune disorder called *Crohn's disease,* as well as a secondary bacterial infection called *C. difficile.*

Mark was in severe pain and discomfort, as you might imagine—a pretty tough haul for a kid! His physicians immediately prescribed 200 mg of prednisone as well as antibiotics and narcotic pain medication. They consulted surgeons, and a daily debate began as to whether they should remove a large portion of Mark's bowels. But they opted to wait and watch Mark's progress over the next few weeks.

Mark slowly improved, and a repeat colonoscopy showed that the infection had cleared. This made the typical ulcerative appearance of Crohn's disease all the more evident. The doctors met with the parents and informed them that this was an incurable autoimmune disease. They explained that for some reason, Mark's immune system had started to attack his own bowels, which created tremendous inflammation and destruction. The team of physicians wanted to place Mark on a chemotherapeutic drug called Imuran, even though he was still taking very high doses of prednisone and narcotic pain medication. Mark started on Imuran, and after a total of six weeks of hospitalization, the boy was delighted to be discharged.

Again, his home stay was a brief one, and within a week Mark was in so much abdominal pain he had to be readmitted to the hospital.

Physicians generally treat patients with autoimmune diseases with drugs that suppress the immune system. Since the body's own immune system is attacking it, it is logical to aggressively quell its activity. But one of the major side effects of these potent drugs is that they wipe out the natural antioxidant defense too. Mark's Crohn's disease was finally coming under control, but his depressed immune system left him vulnerable to all kinds of infections. A cold would turn into a serious pneumonia, and the common flu would put him down for weeks. In fact during the first year after his initial attack on the soccer field, Mark had to be admitted seven times as a result of serious infections. It was about this time that I became involved with the young boy.

Mark's father approached me for my medical advice following a meeting I was speaking at in San Diego and asked what I would recommend. I told him that I'd put Mark on a potent antioxidant and mineral tablet along with high doses of grape-seed extract and CoQ10. I also encouraged his parents to be sure he was getting adequate amounts of the essential fatty acids in his diet or to supplement with a flaxseed oil or fish oil. All of these would restimulate Mark's natural antioxidant defense system.

Mark slowly began to improve but still struggled with abdominal pain and side effects from the drugs. Gradually his doctors took him off prednisone but not the Imuran. Mark's mom and dad consulted me again, and I recommended that they seek a second opinion from a private pediatric gastroenterologist.

After seeing how well Mark was doing aside from Imuran's side effects, the private gastroenterologist felt that it would be well worth trying to get Mark off of all drugs, including the pain medication and Imuran. He was gradually taken off the Imuran, and with the help of a psychologist who taught Mark some relaxation techniques, he was finally able to stop taking all pain medication as well. At last Mark was medication free and felt better than he had since that day of his first attack.

Mark is now doing great and eating a normal diet. I was delighted to see the active fifteen-year-old again recently. What a frightening and painful experience he and his parents endured. A disease that for many offers little hope is manageable for Mark. He is now pain free without having even a flare-up of his Crohn's for more than two and a half years. Needless to say, we are all optimistic about Mark's future.

The lingering question is: How could Mark's immune system turn on him like that? Isn't our immune system supposed to help us? Let's start by looking at how our immune system *should* work.

The Immune System: Our Great Protector

Our immune system guards us against viruses, bacteria, fungi, foreign proteins, and abnormal cancer cells. It is a sophisticated interplay of many different kinds of immune cells. Even though the scope of this book does not allow me to go into much detail about the intricate workings of the immune system, I still believe it is important for you to know who the basic players are. Here is a brief job description of each.

The Different Players in Our Immune System

Macrophages (or phagocytes) are the Pac-Manlike white cells that are the first line of defense. They can quickly attack any foreign invader (virus, bacteria) and actually gobble it up. But sometimes macrophages are not sure if they have attached themselves to a foreign invader or not. They definitely do not want to destroy something that is part of the body (as in Mark's case). This is when they call for help from the T-helper cells.

T-helper cells are from a group of white cells called the *lymphocytes*. A T-helper cell comes along and attaches itself to the macrophage and tries to help it determine if the particle the macrophage has in its grasp is friend or foe. If the T-helper cell determines that it is an enemy, it will secrete hormones called *cytokines* (they stimulate the inflammatory reaction), which literally signal the immune system to kick itself into high gear. This stimulates the B-cells into action and attracts more macrophages and T-helper cells to come to the rescue.

B-cells have the ability to shoot down the intruder with enzymes that destroy it by creating oxidative stress. Some of the B-cells will return to the lymph nodes to create antibodies against these intruders. If this intruder ever shows up again, our immune system is ready for it because of these antibodies.

Natural killer cells can destroy anything in their path. They flood infected cells with toxins and destructive enzymes, which effectively destroys all foreign invaders or cells that are growing abnormally, such as cancer cells.

T-suppressor cells are the riot police that come along after the foreign invader has been destroyed and tries to calm down this tremendous immune response. They are critical for the control of collateral damage. If this highly reactive response goes unchecked, tremendous damage to the surrounding normal tissue could occur. This is what makes the inflammatory response so dangerous. Though it is absolutely necessary to control potential infectious intruders, if the inflammatory response gets out of control, it can cause great harm.

You have already learned that nutritional supplements can significantly enhance the body's natural antioxidant defense. In this chapter you will also begin to realize that these same nutritional supplements can significantly enhance our body's own immune system. Dr. Karlheinz Schmidt stated, "The optimal function of the host defense system depends upon an adequate supply of antioxidant micronutrients."[1] It only makes common sense that if our immune system is going to be able to protect us as God intended, we need to have all the nutrients present at optimal levels.

Nutrients and Our Immune System

Again let's examine the medical literature and see how each of these individual nutrients actually affects our immune response.

Vitamin E

Macrophages that are deficient in vitamin E release more free radicals and do not live as long. Our immune system uses this production of free radicals to destroy these foreign invaders by actually creating oxidative stress. This is the "good" side of oxidative stress as long as it remains under control. Vitamin E deficiency also affects the differentiation of our T-cells in the thymus; this leads to an imbalance of T-helper to T-suppressor cells. The poor production of T-suppressor cells is one of the main reasons that the inflammatory response can get out of hand. Remember that the T-suppressor cells are the riot police that are essential to cooling the immune reaction and so limit collateral damage. Some researchers believe that poor T-suppressor cell function is at the heart of the autoimmune response.[2]

Studies show that supplementation with vitamin E corrects these deficiencies in our immune system and helps clear infections. Clinical studies have also demonstrated that the immune-enhancing effect of vitamin E supplementation was even greater in the elderly and in individuals who had malabsorption syndromes.[3] Mark's disease, for instance, involved both the small bowel and colon, which essentially created a malabsorption of these nutrients. Vitamin E supplementation can also protect against the immunosuppressive effects of cortisol, which is released in great quantities during a stress reaction.

Carotenoids

A well-known property of the carotenoids is the fact that they are capable of protecting the surrounding normal tissue from potential damage created by the inflammatory response of the immune system. Supplementation of the carotenoids can increase the number and effectiveness of the T-helper cells and the natural killer cells, which, as you have already learned, constitutes an important part of our defense system against cancer cells. This greatly improves the tumor surveillance of our immune system.

Vitamin C

Dr. Linus Pauling has been influential in making everyone aware of the importance of supplemental vitamin C and its ability to enhance the immune system. Although we are still arguing whether massive doses of vitamin C are helpful for the common cold, the enhancing effects on the immune system are fairly well established. Vitamin C has been shown to improve the function of the macrophages.[4] This significantly improves the first line of defense against bacterial infections.

It is wiser to take good doses of vitamin C daily rather than massive doses only when you think you are coming down with an infection. In one study those taking 1 g of vitamin C daily for more than two months showed a striking enhancement of several aspects of the immune system. Vitamin C also has the ability to regenerate vitamin E and handle the excessive free radicals within the plasma. Both of these properties further enhance vitamin C's ability to improve the immune system.

Glutathione

Supplementation with the precursors of glutathione (N-acetyl-L-cysteine, selenium, niacin, and vitamin B2) have shown significant enhancement to the overall immune system. Even patients with HIV infections have experienced this positive effect.[5]

Coenzyme Q10

As we age, CoQ10 levels decline and make the mitochondria (the furnace of the cell) especially vulnerable to oxidative damage. CoQ10 is critical for the optimal function of the immune system because of its major role in the production of energy in the cells of the immune system. Supplementation of CoQ10 has been shown to reverse these problems and significantly enhance the immune system.[6]

Zinc

Just about every aspect of our immune system needs zinc. A deficiency actually suppresses several parts of the immune system: the number of lymphocytes decreases, the function of many white cells is severely reduced, and levels of thymic hormone, which is a strong stimulus of the immune system, fall.

Many people reach for their zinc lozenges whenever they get a cold. Studies have shown that taking these lozenges every two hours can shorten the length of a cold by several days. Researchers believe that zinc not only boosts the immune system but also inhibits the replication of the virus.[7] But a word of caution is necessary here: if a person consumes a high dose of zinc for too long, it can actually suppress the immune system. I am not against short-term use of high doses of zinc or even vitamin C with colds; but I believe consistent long-term use of optimal doses of these nutrients in supplementation is better for the antioxidant defense system and the immune system.

When all of the players of our immune system are functioning at their peak capacity, our overall health is obviously the beneficiary. Children are able to optimize their immune system via nutritional supplementation within six months. Aging is generally associated with an impairment of our immune responses, which leads to increased frequency and severity of infections. In fact infections (especially of the respiratory tract) are the fourth most common cause of death in the elderly.[8]

The *British Lancet* recently reported a study in which elderly patients received either optimal levels of nutritional supplements or a placebo. Those patients who received the nutritional supplements had significant improvements of their overall immune response and enjoyed fewer and less severe infections compared to those who received the placebo. It took at least a year of supplementation to optimize their immune systems, but in the end the benefits were dramatic.[9] This study, along with several others, confirms the fact that our immune system is extremely dependent on these micronutrients, as is our antioxidant defense system.

The Inflammatory Response

You have seen throughout this book that inflammation is a serious foe. You understand that heart disease is really an inflammatory disease and not a disease of cholesterol. Mark's devastating problems were all the results of inflammation of the bowel. In Chapter 11 you will read that millions of us are developing arthritis because of increased inflammation in our joints. And the underlying cause of asthma is essentially inflammation.

Simply put, most of us just have too much inflammation in our bodies. We need to bring this excessive inflammation back into balance, and nutritional supplements are the key.

The inflammatory response is the result of a complicated chain of events involving the immune response, which releases tremendous amounts of free radicals, caustic enzymes, and inflammatory cytokines. We have looked at the basic immune response, but we now need to look at how to handle the prolonged inflammatory (chronic inflammation) response that these cytokines create.

Antioxidant supplements are our best tool. They improve our immune system, they help control the inflammatory response, and they build up our antioxidant defense, which in turn protects our normal cells from inflammation's destruction. But there is another important aspect of this inflammatory response we need to look into: our bodies' natural anti-inflammatory system. That's right. Has it ever crossed your mind as you reach for the bottle of Advil that your body makes its own anti-inflammatory products?

Let's take a look at what those products are.

Essential Fatty Acids

Not all fats are bad. In fact an essential fat is just that—essential to the body. The body cannot manufacture these fats and therefore must get them from food. The body uses fats for the production of healthy cell membranes as well as certain hormones called *prostaglandins*. The two most important essential fatty acids are omega-3 fatty acids, called *alpha-linoleic* acid, and omega-6 fatty acids, called just *linoleic acid*. Our bodies turn omega-3 fatty acids into prostaglandins that are primarily anti-inflammatories. Omega-6 fatty acids become prostaglandins that are primarily inflammatories.

The generally accepted optimal ratio of dietary intake of omega-6 fatty acids and omega-3 fatty acids is 4:1. This means we should take in four times as much of omega-6 as we do omega-3.

Omega-6 fatty acids are abundant in the western diet; they are in our meats, dairy products, and processed foods. We get omega-3 fatty acids from vegetable oils such as flaxseed, canola, pumpkin, and soybean oil. These fats are also found in such cold-water fish as mackerel, sardines, salmon, and tuna. As you might guess, the average American consumes a few more omega-6 fatty acids than omega-3s—a lot more, in fact. On average we consume a ratio of 20:1 or even 40:1 of these fats in our diet!

This results in our bodies producing *significantly* more inflammatory products than anti-inflammatory products. Our bodies are simply too inflamed. The imbalance in the consumption of these essential fatty acids is the main reason for the imbalance in our body's production of these hormones. That is why many individuals in the industrialized world need to take flaxseed oil and fish oil in supplementation in an attempt to bring these back into balance.

Here is another unknown fact: essential fats also have the ability to actually decrease our total cholesterol levels and our LDL (bad) cholesterol levels. This means that not all fats are created equal. I not only encourage my patients to supplement the omega-3 fatty acids but also to decrease their intake of saturated fat. When you combine these two efforts, the inflammation in the body readily comes back under control and your cholesterol levels improve.

Several studies have shown significant clinical improvements in patients with rheumatoid arthritis, lupus, heart disease, multiple sclerosis, and almost any disease that involves inflammation when they consume these important essential fats in supplementation.[10] This is a very important aspect of maintaining your health or redeeming your health if you have already lost it.

We have looked at various aspects of our immune system and how it is supposed to work. We have also looked at the problem when this normal inflammatory response gets carried away. But now we need to look at the very worst scenario—what happens when our immune system mounts a mutiny and actually starts to attack our own body.

Autoimmune Diseases

You've heard the saying: "One's greatest strength is also his greatest weakness." This is no truer than in the immune system. Many clinicians believe that every disease is essentially the result of a breakdown of our immune system. But in the bizarre case of autoimmune disease, the immune system actually becomes the body's worst enemy itself by attacking normal cells and tissue. If it attacks the joint space, we call it rheumatoid arthritis; if it attacks our bowels, we call it Crohn's disease or ulcerative colitis; if it attacks the myelin sheath of our nerves, we call it multiple sclerosis; and when it attacks the connective tissue of our body, we call it lupus or scleroderma.

Why and how does this happen? I learned in medical school that autoimmune diseases were the result of an "overactive" immune system that begins attacking "self" instead of "nonself." But it made more sense to me that in the case of autoimmune disease, the immune system, rather than being overactive, had instead become *confused* and was now attacking the body rather than foreign invaders as it was designed to do.

In a recent review article on autoimmune diseases reported in the *New England Journal of Medicine*, the authors pointed out that no one really knows for certain *why* the immune system literally turns on "self." But many researchers not only believe that oxidative stress is the underlying cause of every autoimmune disease, but that it also could be the culprit that causes our immune system to actually attack us.[11]

Several studies have documented the fact that the root cause of autoimmune diseases is oxidative stress.[12] As you may anticipate, the antioxidant levels in persons with rheumatoid arthritis, lupus, MS, Crohn's, and scleroderma are significantly decreased. Low antioxidant levels have also been shown to increase one's risk of developing rheumatoid arthritis or lupus. The clinical indicators of oxidative stress are also very high in these patients, especially during a flare-up period of these diseases.[13]

Antioxidant supplementation would therefore be ideal for patients with these autoimmune diseases. Not only can antioxidant supplements optimize the natural antioxidant defense system, but they also can enhance our immune system and help control the inflammatory response. In other words they can help bring oxidative stress back under control and circumvent this entire vicious cycle.

Matt's Story

Matt is a successful lawyer in the Chicago area, which basically means he has worked long, hard hours to build his practice while working equally hard to balance his priorities of wife and family. His health had always been good, so he never thought much about it until the fall of 1996.

Matt was attending a wedding when he began to feel some significant abdominal discomfort. He had been extremely busy the two weeks prior to the wedding, so he thought he might be coming down with a flu bug. A day or so later, he felt like he'd been "hit by a Mack truck," as he put it, he was so fatigued with body aches.

When his symptoms worsened, Matt decided to go to the doctor. By this point he was experiencing waves of severe abdominal pain. Desperate for relief, he asked the doctor to take out whatever was causing the pain. He underwent all kinds of tests, including CT scans, ultrasounds, x-rays, and numerous blood tests. So you can imagine Matt's shock when no diagnosis became apparent. He was sent home with only a painkiller.

Matt had recently been reading about nutritional supplementation and decided to start an aggressive supplement program. But he did not improve very much. He still felt miserable. He felt achy all over, and he remained extremely fatigued. He finally saw a specialist who ordered a blood test called

ANA (antinuclear antibody). Matt's ANA came back positive at a level of 1:640 (normal is 1:40 or less). His specialist told him that he had systemic lupus erythematosus, or what most people simply refer to as lupus.

The ANA was an indicator of an autoimmune process gone amuck. His body's immune system was actually attacking itself. Once Matt heard this, he increased his supplements even more and started taking 350 mg of grapeseed extract along with his antioxidants and minerals. He slowly improved and required less and less pain medication, even though he still had intermittent bouts of pain. The process was long and hard as Matt continued to fight fatigue and the flulike symptoms.

By January Matt was feeling much better and was able to make up for lost time by getting back to working ten-hour days. He was thrilled because he had not been able to work at all for about four months. Being able to support his family financially was something Matt was not sure would ever be possible again.

When he went back for a follow-up visit several months later, his specialist wanted to start him on some chemotherapeutic drugs, a standard treatment for lupus. Needless to say, Matt insisted that he felt great and was not having any problems. When his specialist looked at his repeat ANA report, his jaw dropped. He couldn't believe it.

"Matt, your ANA has crashed!" he exclaimed. "It's now only 1:40 and is basically normal." He congratulated Matt and encouraged him to just keep taking whatever medication his doctor had put him on. When Matt informed him that he wasn't taking any medication, the specialist replied, "I don't know what you are doing, but keep it up."

Matt continues to do well. He's not been sick for more than five years now and his ANA tests remain negative. In fact he claims that he feels better now than he felt before he contracted lupus. Though he realizes it's not true, Matt doesn't feel like he has lupus anymore. Its symptoms may return, and they might not. No one can say for sure. But one thing is certain: Matt will never take his health for granted again.

•   •   •

The important aspect in Matt's story was the fact that he started this aggressive nutritional supplement program early in the course of his disease. I have presented a number of clinical stories in which patients were actually able to redeem their health after their disease had progressed fairly significantly. I hope that more and more people will start to supplement their diet before they even get sick, and then become more aggressive with optimizers as soon as they realize they have a major illness. A supplement program can't hurt—it can only help. (For detailed information on starting supplementation, see Chapter 17.)

ELEVEN | Arthritis and Osteoporosis

HOW DOES THE OLD SAYING GO? WE ALL CAN COUNT ON TWO things in life: death and taxes. As I write this chapter, I groan with new awareness of the quickly approaching tax deadline. But I'm also reminded of a third thing most all of us can count on in life—arthritis. It's true: approximately 70 to 80 percent of people in the U.S. over fifty years of age suffer to some extent with the most common type of arthritis called *osteoarthritis*, also known as *degenerative arthritis*.[1]

You are probably much too familiar with the symptoms of early morning stiffness, mildly swollen joints, and joint pain. Osteoarthritis is by far the most common chronic degenerative disease that I see in my office. Affecting men and women alike, it can involve every joint in the body, including the neck and lower back. As arthritis gets worse, it can cause significant discomfort, pain, and even disability.

Osteoarthritis is mainly a degeneration of the cartilage in the joints. But it can also involve the synovial lining (the lining of the joint) and the underlying bone. As the joint cartilage begins to wear down, it causes increased stress to the bone. In response to this intensified stress, the bone actually becomes denser. It is very common to see bone spurs forming around the joint as a result.

You may have heard a family member or friend say he needs to have a joint replaced because he has "bone on bone." What he is really saying is that the cartilage (the cushion) of his joint is entirely gone. Since degenerative arthritis primarily involves the weight-bearing joints (hips and knees), repeated mechanical stress caused by excessive weight, trauma, or activity is a contributor to the development and progression of this disease.

How Is the Joint Actually Damaged?

Articular cartilage covers the ends of our bones, while joints like the knees also have additional cartilage that acts as a cushion between the bones. Cartilage is primarily made up of collagen fibers, glycoproteins, and proteoglycans. The structural integrity of human cartilage is continually going through a cycle of building up and breaking down. In other words, our bodies need to be building cartilage at the same rate as it's wearing down in order to maintain healthy joints. Again, a balance is the key. When a joint begins to wear out, we know that either the breakdown of cartilage has increased or the production of cartilage has decreased.

That osteoarthritis is an inflammatory disease is a well-known fact. If you observe anyone with arthritic hands, you can actually see how inflamed and swollen the joints of the fingers and hands become. Have you ever wondered what exactly is causing the inflammation and how this leads to damage of the cartilage? The answer is a multifaceted one, because there are actually several sources for inflammation that occur within the joint, as you can see in the box below.

Causes of Inflammation in Our Joints

Cytokines are some of the leading causes of joint inflammation. These proteins carry messages between cells and regulate immunity and inflammation. Two of the most important cytokines are tumor necrosis factor alpha (TNF-a) and interleukin one beta (IL-1B). These are highly concentrated in the joints of people who have osteoarthritis.

Proteases, enzymes that cause the breakdown of proteins, also have been shown to create inflammation in the joint. Proteases are under the control of the cytokines. Some have anti-inflammatory qualities, and some have pro-inflammatory (inflammation-creating) qualities. Obviously, in arthritis the pro-inflammatory proteases are winning.

Phagocytes (neutrophils) are attracted to the inflamed joint in an attempt to clear this reaction and prevent damage to the cartilage and synovial lining. But as you have just learned in the last chapter, this inflammatory response is not always a good thing. Neutrophils can actually lead to more inflammation in the joint.

The *ischemia-reperfusion phenomenon* is a process that sounds difficult but actually is simple. As we use a weight-bearing joint like a hip or knee, the pressure created by our weight when we walk, or especially when we run, blocks the blood flow to the cartilage. This is known as *ischemia* or lack of blood supply. When we take our weight off the joint, the pressure lessens and blood is allowed to return to the cartilage (this is called *reperfusion*). This process, as well as the sources of inflammation I've just listed, causes excessive production of free radicals. In turn, the free radicals heavily tax the antioxidant defense system and cause oxidative stress.

When the antioxidant defense system is overwhelmed, oxidative stress within the joint causes damage to the cartilage and synovial lining of the joint. When the body cannot rebuild cartilage fast enough, the joint begins to deteriorate.

Another Arthritis: Rheumatoid

Rheumatoid arthritis is an autoimmune disease (see Chapter 10). This occurs when the immune system begins attacking the cartilage and the synovial lining of the joint. As a result, an unbalanced (i.e., unhealthy) inflammatory process begins significant destruction of healthy tissue. Not only does this inflammatory response create excessive free radicals, it also attracts cytokines, especially TNF-a.

Studies show that TNF-a is extremely high in the plasma of patients with rheumatoid arthritis. Studies also indicate that free-radical production is five times higher in rheumatoid arthritis patients when compared to patients with normal joints.[2] Thus tremendous oxidative stress is at work, causing damage to the joints in those suffering with rheumatoid arthritis.

If you know anyone who suffers from rheumatoid arthritis, you are well aware of how damaging this disease is; it often causes incapacitating deformity and pain. Though people with rheumatoid arthritis have significantly greater oxidative stress than those with osteoarthritis, the destruction of the cartilage in both of these diseases arises from oxidative stress. It is important to understand the underlying causes of these diseases as you consider now the traditional treatments offered in medicine.[3]

Traditional Treatment of Arthritis

The basic traditional treatment of both osteoarthritis and rheumatoid arthritis is the use of nonsteroidal anti-inflammatories (NSAIDS) and aspirin. While these drugs reduce inflammation in joints, they are also responsible for the frequent adverse side effects of stomach ulcers and upper-gastrointestinal (GI) bleeding. In fact more than one hundred thousand admissions to hospitals in the U.S. per year and more than sixteen thousand deaths each year are the result of upper-GI bleeding caused by the use of NSAIDS.

In response to the dangerous effects of these NSAIDS, pharmaceutical companies have developed a group of new NSAIDS that primarily block just the COX-2 enzymes. Drugs called COX-2 inhibitors arrived on the market with great fanfare because they caused significantly less GI side effects. Unfortunately, these have side effects as well, including bowel perforation as well as upper GI bleeds although not nearly as frequent as the first generation NSAIDS.

My greatest concern regarding the tremendous use of NSAIDS by arthritis patients is the fact that these drugs merely provide pain relief without attacking the underlying cause of the disease—oxidative stress. Patients with severe rheumatoid arthritis are also being treated with more potent anti-inflammatory drugs like prednisone and gold or chemotherapeutic drugs like methotrexate or Imuran.

Peggie's Story

Peggie is an attractive lady I've had the pleasure of knowing over the past several years. When I first met Peggie, her lower leg was actually angled to the outside because her knee had degenerated so significantly. She was not only having a lot of discomfort in her knee but also in her right hip because she had to walk at a difficult angle.

Peggie talked to me about the tremendous degenerative arthritis that had developed in her right knee following a skiing accident that occurred when she was a teenager. The accident had damaged the cartilage in her knee, and then a short time later she reinjured it. After the second injury she had no choice but to have an operation, and the surgeon removed a major portion of seriously damaged cartilage. In spite of doing all he could, her doctor warned her that she would have a lot of problems with her knee in the future.

Her specialist had given her a brace to wear over her right knee to protect it primarily when she was active. The only other thing he advised her to do was keep the pain under control by using NSAIDS and delay having a knee replacement as long as possible. Peggie knew that a joint replacement would last only somewhere between eight and twelve years, if she was lucky. Being so young, she had four or five times that many years left to live. What should she do?

When I met Peggie, her doctors had discussed the knee-replacement option with her, and she was strongly considering it. The longer she delayed the surgery, the better, but she had to weigh the pain of her current situation with the prognosis of her future.

Peggie determined to do all she could to postpone surgery but not at the expense of her quality of life. She had read a great deal about supplementation and believed an aggressive nutritional supplement program would make a better quality of life possible for her. She began taking a potent antioxidant and mineral combination along with some grape-seed extract, essential fatty acids, calcium, and magnesium supplements. She also started taking 2,000 mg of glucosamine sulfate.

Peggie continued following her physical therapy guidelines and ate a balanced diet. Within a few months of beginning a nutritional supplement program, Peggie could already begin to feel and see improvement. She was less dependent on her NSAIDS and was now able to do more than she had for years. She became much more active and felt less pain. In fact she even overcame her fears and went snow skiing for the first time in years.

Most exciting for Peggie, however, was when she returned to her physician and had repeat x-rays taken of her knee. Her physician was amazed when he compared the current x-rays to those taken two years prior. The comparison revealed that her leg was not angled as much, and he could see increased separation of her bones. Pointing this out to Peggie, he explained that the increased separation of bone on her knee x-ray was evidence that the cartilage had grown back.

Peggie was not altogether surprised at these findings because she could feel the difference and had learned about this possibility during her research on nutritional medicine. The documented improvement from her doctor was just the icing on the cake.

Peggie continues to be active and does pretty much everything she desires to do (she still wears a knee brace for any aggressive sports), and she continues to take supplements. She celebrates each year as one more she has delayed a joint replacement.

Why is Peggie doing so well? Let's look at the strategy she pursued. Peggie first determined to fully understand the underlying problem—at the cellular level—of the degenerative arthritis that followed her accidents. She did this through individual study and by attending scientific meetings. Second, she considered all the possible solutions available, and third, she put her knowledge into action.

Antioxidant Supplements

Like Peggie, anyone who is suffering from degenerative arthritis needs to take a potent, well-balanced antioxidant and mineral supplement. Strong evidence exists that patients who suffer from arthritis are deficient in several antioxidants and supporting nutrients such as vitamin D, vitamin C, vitamin E, boron (a mineral), and vitamin B3.[4] As you have been learning throughout this book, you need to supply all these antioxidants at optimal levels in an attempt to bring oxidative stress under control.

Peggie was taking all of these nutrients in supplementation, as well as another important one: glucosamine sulfate.

Glucosamine Sulfate

Glucosamine is one of the basic nutrients for the synthesis of cartilage. It is a simple amino sugar that is the primary building block of proteoglycans, which are the molecules that give cartilage its elasticity. Unlike NSAIDS and aspirin, glucosamine does not simply cover up the pain but rather helps to rebuild the damaged cartilage. Early studies showed short-term benefits of the use of glucosamine sulfate; however, most physicians remained unimpressed.[5]

In 1999 a three-year, large, randomized-sample, placebo-controlled, double-blind clinical trial (the sort of studies doctors really like) was reported at the Annual Meeting of the American College of Rheumatology. This study showed that glucosamine not only reduced the pain and inflammation of arthritis but actually stopped the deterioration of the cartilage. What was even more impressive was the fact that there was evidence of actual cartilage regrowth—just as in Peggie's case. The placebo group members, who took the traditional NSAIDS, continued to experience rapid deterioration of their joints.[6]

This study, along with several others, has shown the significant health benefit for arthritis patients who take glucosamine sulfate supplements in the 1,500–2,000-mg range, with virtually no side effects. Even more exciting is the fact that when the patients in the clinical trial discontinued their glucosamine, the pain did not return for weeks and even months later.[7]

NSAIDS, on the other hand, have significant side effects such as ulcers, upper GI bleeding, and possible liver damage, as I noted earlier. Considering that these drugs do absolutely nothing to slow down the degenerative process and in fact may accelerate it, we must wonder why NSAIDS are some of the most prescribed medications in the world. To the dismay of pharmaceutical companies, more and more physicians are recommending glucosamine sulfate to their patients.

The results I have seen in my practice are impressive. Even though I recommend glucosamine to all my arthritis patients, I also prescribe NSAIDS for quick relief. It is exciting to discover my patients who decide to take glucosamine eventually hardly ever need to take their NSAIDS. When they are willing to add the antioxidants, minerals, essential fats, and grape-seed extract, they do even better.

I'm not alone in my convictions. Many of my orthopedic friends support the use of glucosamine too, since they realize that being able to delay a joint replacement is ultimately in the patient's best interest.

Chondroitin Sulfate

Chondroitin sulfate is often combined with glucosamine sulfate to create a one-two punch. Chondroitin makes up part of the proteoglycans and is responsible for attracting water into the cartilage. This makes the cartilage more pliable and spongy. Without this important nutrient the cartilage becomes drier and more fragile.

I personally feel that the most important nutrient is still glucosamine sulfate. Oral chondroitin needs to be studied more thoroughly in larger number of patients, allowing more plausible evidence as to whether chondroitin is really a player or not. I also believe MSM (a natural anti-inflammatory) needs to be studied more thoroughly. But I have had several patients who experienced a significant response when they added it to their regime.

Chondroitin Sulfate

Several studies show improvement in patients with arthritis who are getting additional chondroitin. But many of these positive studies have involved actual IV injections of chondroitin, and some researchers are concerned that chondroitin is not effectively absorbed through the GI tract. Some say that it is broken down, then absorbed, and reassembled within the joint cartilage. I feel further studies are needed to determine its overall importance in the treatment of osteoarthritis.[8]

Osteoporosis

Osteoporosis is a nutritional deficiency at literally epidemic proportions in the U.S. In one of the richest, most well-fed nations of the world, more than 25 million Americans are living with the crippling effects of osteoporosis at a cost of about $14 billion each year to the U.S. economy. At least 1.2 million fractures occur each year in the United States as a direct result of osteoporosis.[9] I have actually seen patients fracture hips as they simply walked into my office, without any kind of fall or injury. Spontaneous compression fractures of the vertebrae and of the back cause tremendous pain and suffering in my patients with osteoporosis.

Osteoporosis has been presented to the American public as a disease merely dependent on estrogen and calcium. In response to this national crisis, the health-care community is treating menopausal women with Hormonal Replacement Therapy (HRT) in an effort to curb any onset of osteoporosis.

Although many believe that HRT can slow the progression of osteoporosis, it may do more harm than good. In 1997 the *New England Journal of Medicine* reviewed several studies involving women who took estrogen replacement for more than five to ten years. The results shocked reviewers, revealing more than a 40 percent increase in breast cancer. The pharmaceutical companies quickly responded to this negative report by convincing the doctors that the benefits of HRT far outweighed the risks, often boasting that other clinical trials had shown that patients who took HRT decreased their risk of heart attacks, strokes, and Alzheimer's dementia.[10]

Two other major studies, however, the Heart and Estrogen/Progestin

Replacement Study (HERS) and The Women's Health Initiative Study, did not show any slowing of the progression of heart disease. In fact some evidence suggested that the patients taking HRT had an *increase* in the incidence of heart attacks, especially in the first year. Interestingly, these studies did show that those taking HRT experienced a significant decrease in LDL (bad) cholesterol and a significant increase in HDL (good) cholesterol. So why did these patients have an increased risk of heart disease?

I believe the answer appeared in other studies that have shown women who take synthetic HRT had a tremendous increase in their C-reactive proteins, which you may recall is a measure of the inflammation in the artery. It is a much better predictor of future heart attacks than is cholesterol—especially in women. Remember, heart disease is an inflammatory disease of the artery, not a disease of cholesterol.

When women who want to avoid osteoporosis consider synthetic Hormonal Replacement Therapy in light of these new clinical studies, perhaps the good does not outweigh the bad—especially when you consider the well-known increased risk of developing blood clots in the legs and gall bladder disease in those patients taking HRT. Several new drugs have arrived on the market for osteoporosis, such as Fosomax, Actonel, Evista, and Calcitonin, which have the ability to actually increase bone density. Doctors are recommending these drugs more and more instead of HRT, primarily because of the growing concern over the adverse effects of long-term HRT therapy. Short-term studies using these drugs have demonstrated a significantly decreased risk of fractures and repeat fractures.[11] For a thorough discussion about these and other problems women face during their menopausal time, I recommend Dr. Christiane Northrup's book, entitled *The Wisdom of Menopause*.

Not Just Calcium—Bones Are Living Tissue

Remember Mr. Bones, the skeleton that graced the back of the biology room in high school and college? He was the lead character in many a great prank as well as the main player on the comprehensive exam. Though the popular plastic model has taught lots of kids about bones, we often think of "bare bones" (like his) instead of bone that is active, living tissue, which is continually remodeling itself through osteoblastic (bone forming) and osteoclastic (bone resorbing) activity.

Bone is not just a collection of calcium crystals; rather it is living tissue constantly engaged in biochemical reactions that are dependent on many different micronutrients and enzyme systems. Therefore, like any living tissue, bone has diverse nutritional needs.

The American diet, with its high intake of white breads, white flour, refined sugars, and fat, is terribly deficient in many of these essential nutrients. Our nation's diet is also high in meats and carbonated beverages, which increase the intake of phosphorous and decrease our absorption of calcium. Inadequate intake of any nutrients required for bone health contributes to osteoporosis.

Another common myth that teams up with Mr. Bare Bones is that calcium is all we need for strong bones and to stave off osteoporosis. But the truth is that a variety of essential nutrients must be present, not just calcium, to have any success in decreasing the amount of osteoporosis in this country.

In order to reduce the risk of fractures of the spine, hip, and wrist, we must pay attention to several important factors: preserving adequate bone mass, preventing the loss of the protein matrix part of the bone, and making sure that the bone has all the proper nutrients it needs to repair and replace damaged areas of bone. Nutritional supplementation plays a vital role in all three areas of preserving and building bone.

Let's take a look at each nutrient and how it aids in the fight against osteoporosis.

Calcium

There is no doubt that calcium deficiency can lead to osteoporosis. But studies show skeletal calcium depletion in only 25 percent of postmenopausal women. Indeed, calcium supplements in these women did seem to increase bone mass, but the supplements had no effect on the other 75 percent who were not calcium deficient. Recent studies of calcium and vitamin D supplementation present a *slowing down* of osteoporosis but in no way demonstrate that supplementation *prevented* it. These studies have also shown a reduction in fractures of the hip, spine, and wrist.[12] In other words calcium is helpful, but it isn't *the* answer.

Calcium is an essential nutrient in the fight against osteoporosis. Both men and women should take supplements of 800–1,500 mg daily, depending on the amount of calcium they are getting in their diet. People more consistently absorb calcium citrate than calcium carbonate; but when taken with food and good levels of vitamin D, the absorption level is quite similar.

Whatever form of calcium you take, you should consume it with food for optimal absorption.

Be advised that children also need this level of supplementation. In fact studies prove that children who take 800–1,200 mg of calcium daily prior to puberty will increase their bone density by 5–7 percent. This finding is significant because this increase in their bone density will carry over as they develop into young adults and throughout their lifetimes.[13]

Magnesium

Magnesium is important in several biochemical reactions that take place within the bone. Magnesium activates alkaline phosphatase, which is a required enzyme in the process of forming new bone crystals. And vitamin D needs magnesium to convert to its most active form. If there is a deficiency in magnesium, it can lead to a syndrome of vitamin D resistance.

Dietary surveys have shown 80 to 85 percent of Americans consume a magnesium-deficient diet.[14]

Vitamin D

Vitamin D is necessary for the absorption of calcium. Vitamin D is typically produced in the skin when it is exposed to sunlight. But as you know, with age people tend to spend less time in the sun, and vitamin D deficiencies become very common.

We also take in vitamin D orally via fortified foods and milk, but it must then be converted to its biologically active form, vitamin D3. Often the impaired conversion of vitamin D to vitamin D3 may be more of a problem than deficient intake. This is why I recommend supplementation of vitamin D by using the active form, D3.

The *New England Journal of Medicine* reported a study in which researchers looked at the level of vitamin D in 290 consecutive patients admitted to the medical ward of Massachusetts General Hospital. These were patients who had been normally active and were not admitted from a nursing home. Hospital staff checked their vitamin D levels and found that 93 percent were deficient. Surprisingly, those patients who were taking a multiple vitamin were also deficient in their vitamin D levels 93 percent of the time. This finding is critical when you realize that you don't absorb any calcium without vitamin D!

The study concluded by stating that *everyone* should be taking vitamin D supplements and at a level significantly higher than the recommended daily allowance. In fact the researchers concluded that supplementing with 500–800 IU of vitamin D daily is critical if we are going to have any effect on the epidemic of osteoporosis.[15] And remember—you will absorb calcium much better if you take it along with vitamin D and food.

Vitamin K

Vitamin K is required to synthesize osteocalcin, a protein found in large quantities within the bone. It is therefore critical in bone formation, remodeling, and repair. In a clinical trial supplementing vitamin K in patients with osteoporosis reduced urinary calcium loss by 18 to 50 percent. This means vitamin K helps the body absorb and retain calcium rather than excrete it.[16]

Manganese

Manganese is necessary for the synthesis of connective tissue in cartilage and bone. Like magnesium, manganese is lost in the processing of whole grains into refined flour. A study of osteoporotic women showed their manganese levels were only 25 percent of those of the women in the control group.[17] This nutrient also needs to be present at optimal levels if you have any desire to prevent osteoporosis.

Folic Acid, Vitamin B6, and Vitamin B12

Does this combination sound familiar? It should. Homocysteine (see Chapter 6) is not only bad for your blood vessels, but it is also bad for your bones. Individuals with severe elevations of homocysteine have been found to have significant osteoporosis as well.

Interestingly, *pre*menopausal women have greater efficiency in breaking down methionine and thus have little buildup of homocysteine. This changes dramatically after menopause. Postmenopausal women have much higher levels of homocysteine. Could this explain in part both the increased risk of heart disease and osteoporosis in postmenopausal women?[18] The fact remains these women need higher amounts of folic acid, vitamin B6, and vitamin B12.

Boron

Boron is an interesting nutrient when it comes to bone metabolism. When study subjects took boron in supplementation, the urinary excretion of calcium decreased by approximately 40 percent. Boron also increases magnesium concentrations and decreases phosphorous levels.[19] Supplementation with 3 mg daily of boron is more than adequate.

Silicon

Silicon is important because of its ability to strengthen the connective tissue matrix, which strengthens bone. Patients with osteoporosis, in whom the generation of new bone is desirable, need increased amounts of silicon.

Zinc

This mineral is essential for the normal functioning of vitamin D. Low serum zinc levels were found in the serum and bones of patients with osteoporosis.[20]

Prevention of Osteoporosis

I promise you this: you do not want to get osteoporosis. I have treated several patients suffering from severe cases. It is a debilitating, painful disease. They seem to suffer continual fractures of the spine and are in extreme pain for long periods of time. As I've mapped out, osteoporosis is not simply a disease arising from a lack of calcium and estrogen. Our bodies need multiple nutrients for bone remodeling and the production of good healthy bone.

We also need to control our oxidative stress. Recent studies demonstrate that people with decreased bone density have increased oxidative stress. So you not only want to supplement with these important nutrients needed for bone production, but also take all of the antioxidants and supporting nutrients to build up your antioxidant defense system.

I encourage all my patients, both women and men, preferably before they reach forty years of age, to begin supplementation with a high-quality antioxidant and mineral tablets along with additional amounts of calcium, magnesium, boron, and silicon. It is critical for adults also to eat a healthy diet and develop a modest exercise program. Weight-bearing exercises need to be part of the program as they are a necessary component in stimulating the body to make more bone. Walking may help the lower legs but does very little for the back and hips; upper body weight resistance exercises such as lifting weights over your head are critical to anyone who is trying to protect herself or himself from this devastating disease.

Even when my menopausal patients find out they have evidence of early thinning of the bone, called *osteopenia,* they usually find that they can improve their bone density with this same program. I postpone prescribing drugs like Fosomax, Actonel, Evista, or Calcitonin in this situation if my patients are willing to make some lifestyle changes: taking these high-quality supplements, along with eating an improved diet and using a weight-bearing exercise program.

I follow these patients closely by repeating their DEXA (bone density) scan in one year. If they are stable or improving, I keep them on their program and continue to follow them closely. If they experience more thinning of their bones, I will start them on one of these newer drugs.

• • •

The key to both preventing arthritis and osteoporosis is cellular nutrition. I have presented several individual nutrients here to give you a glimpse of what the medical literature is telling us about their importance.

As you've seen, preventing these potentially crippling conditions is not simply a matter of boosting a calcium or estrogen deficiency. This is just one more area in which nutritional supplements work with your body to maintain the health you have or regain that which you have lost.

TWELVE | Lung Disease

THE YOUNG MOTHER SLEEPILY OPENED THE DOOR INTO HER toddler's bedroom to check one last time on two-year-old Christian before she went to bed. As she bent down to kiss his forehead, sheer terror overcame her: her son was blue and not breathing.

After calling 911 she began trying to resuscitate him. The paramedics arrived and moments later Christian was in transit to the emergency room. They continued to perform cardiopulmonary resuscitation because the little boy's heart had stopped beating. But only the ER doctor was successful in getting Christian's heart and lungs to respond.

The once-lively little boy was admitted to the hospital with the diagnosis of severe asthma.

The doctors stabilized Christian and started him on a drug called *theophylline* which dilates the airways. Though his parents were relieved that Christian had survived, they were terrified about his future—they had had no idea asthma could manifest itself so suddenly or become so severe. Obviously motivated to be sure Christian received all of his medication, his parents took the fragile boy home.

Minimal lung reserve marred Christian's childhood. He could not participate in normal rambunctious activities with the other children, and as he grew older, the doctors kept adding more and more medication because his lungs were just not performing well.

Then when Christian was age fifteen, it happened again. He experienced another severe asthmatic attack. Passing out at home, he quit breathing. Again, with flashbacks from the past, his parents called the paramedics as they attempted to resuscitate their son. His heart and lungs finally responded only after the family reached the ER. After this hospital admission Christian was placed on the anti-inflammatory drug prednisone, which he would continue to take for the next fourteen years.

At the age of twenty-seven, with very little lung function left, Christian was taking nine different drugs. His pulmonary function tests showed that his large airways were working at only 17 percent of normal capacity while his small airways were working at a mere 8 percent. In spite of all his medication, Christian was barely able to live his life. Unable to do anything requiring physical exertion, he lived with the residing fear of having another acute asthmatic attack. He had to continually make sure he had his inhalers and backups with plenty of medication. His life depended on them.

It was at this time that Christian decided to try building his body up by taking a potent antioxidant and mineral tablet with each meal. Within ninety days Christian could tell he was doing better. Because of these encouraging results, he began taking some additional vitamin C, calcium, magnesium, and grape-seed extract. Over the next twenty months, Christian's lung function improved enough that his doctor finally took him off the prednisone. Christian once said to me, "A person should only be on prednisone fourteen days—not fourteen years!"

Christian's repeated pulmonary function tests showed consistent, significant improvement. After being on the supplement program for two years, Christian found that his large airways were working at 87 percent of normal capacity and his small airways were working at 56 percent—not bad considering he had decreased the number of medications he was taking from nine to three during this same time period.

His Albuterol inhaler used to last only one month. Now it lasts at least six months, and half the time he doesn't even know where it is. Today Christian is able to participate in sports and exercise comfortably. His asthma is simply not controlling his life anymore.

Lungs and Air Pollution

When you consider the major causes of oxidative stress in the body, the most serious and the most potent causes enter the body through the respiratory tract. This begins with the nasal passageways and ends with the very thin-lined alveoli of the lung. The air that we breathe today is filled with ozone, nitrogen oxides, fuel emissions, and secondary cigarette smoke. In short: breathe in, cough out.

I will never forget my long journey to San Diego to start my internship at Mercy Hospital. I stopped along the way to see friends in Azusa. The smog was unbelievable, especially for a small-town boy from South Dakota. The next morning my friend took me outside in his yard to look at the magnificent San Bernardino Mountains. There was only one problem: we could not see them. I will never forget when he took a deep breath and told me how great the fresh morning air felt.

I took a deep breath and couldn't stop coughing. In fact later that day I was out playing a round of golf and every time I took a breath I coughed. After about the seventh hole, I had to quit. I was embarrassed because I couldn't even stop coughing when the other players were trying to hit their shots or putt. Anyone who knows me knows how much I love to play golf. For me to quit in the middle of a round of golf, it had to be bad!

It was odd to hear locals in Azusa joke about not trusting air they couldn't see. This was my introduction to what the news later reported as a *moderate* smog day.

Air pollutants cause a tremendous amount of oxidative stress in the respiratory tract and in turn, the body. When you add the most potent cause of oxidative stress to the body—cigarette smoking—you put your nasal passageways and lungs literally under attack.

Still, God did not leave us defenseless. He created a sophisticated and elaborate defense system against this attack on our respiratory system.

The Natural Protection of the Lung

The first line of defense against these poisonous pro-oxidants is called the *epithelial lining fluids* (ELFs). From your nose to the tip of your lungs, the cells are covered with a thick mucous lining. The epithelial cells themselves have cilia, which form a very fine brush border. This brush border sweeps the inhaled foreign particles, bacteria, and viruses back outside. The thick mucous lining contains many antioxidants that then neutralize the inhaled pollutants like ozone, nitrogen dioxide, and fuel emissions. They provide a layer of protection that is so effective that most of the time these pollutants don't even come in contact with the underlying epithelial cells.

With ELFs as the first line of defense, the mucous, cilia, and immune response form a team that is extraordinarily effective in preventing infections in the respiratory tract. The underlying epithelial cells actually produce and secrete several antioxidants into this mucous barrier, including vitamin C, vitamin E, and glutathione. All of these work hard to neutralize all the pollutants we inhale and thus protect the underlying lung tissue and lung function. Vitamin C is the most prominent antioxidant in this protective fluid lining. It is not only an important antioxidant in this fluid but also has the ability to regenerate vitamin E and glutathione.

Still, respiratory tract infections or exposure to airborne pollutants can overwhelm these local antibacteria, antiviral, and antioxidant systems found in the epithelial lining fluids (ELFs). When this happens, a tremendous inflammatory-immune response occurs. The fluids in the lining of the lungs become very thick as the immune response attracts in many white cells that literally attack the invading organisms or pollutants.

As you have learned already, our immune response can cause an exaggerated amount of inflammation. If the invaders are quickly cleared out, everything settles down. But an inability to terminate or control the inflammatory response can result in injury to the underlying epithelial cells. This in turn can lead to chronic inflammation that can cause marked damage to the lung tissue and impair function.

Asthma

This chronic inflammation in the lung causes significant fatigue and a depleted immune system. Whether the immune system is fighting a chronic infection or pollutants in the air, chronic inflammation takes its toll on asthmatics, especially children. Kids seem to continually fight one infection after another, and their energy level is nowhere near that of children with healthy airways.

When I first began my private practice in the early 1970s, physicians believed the underlying problem with asthma was bronchospasm. This is a condition in which the circular muscles surrounding our airway tubes actually go into spasm and narrow the passageways of our lungs, resulting in a very tight feeling in the chest, shortness of breath, and wheezing (usually loud enough to hear without a stethoscope). Our first line of therapy back then was to use drugs like theophylline or Albuterol, which primarily worked on relieving the bronchospasm. If the person was in serious trouble or even had to be admitted to the hospital, we would then add a potent anti-inflammatory medication called *prednisone*.

After a few years into my practice, however, research started to reveal that the underlying problem with asthma was a chronic inflammatory response. Our therapies changed considerably, and we shelved the theophylline-like drugs in favor of anti-inflammatory drugs (inhaled steroids or Intal) as first-line therapy. Research conducted over the past decade has since deduced that the underlying cause of asthma, and most every chronic lung disease, is the result of oxidative stress.[1]

My children's physical education teacher told me that when she began teaching twenty years ago she would ask the school kids to run a mile. It was no big deal. Now the story is altogether different. When she asks kids to run a mile, she ends up with two pockets full of inhalers. Asthma is literally an epidemic in our children across the U.S. and the industrialized world.

When I spoke in London and the Netherlands, the greatest concern of the audience members was the severity of asthma present in their children. I've found that our current generation of children worldwide is exposed to more airborne pollutants than any previous generation. I see children who haven't even reached two years of age who are suffering from serious asthma. The amount of drugs children are taking just so they can breathe is mind-boggling.

Most drugs are now aimed at decreasing this inflammatory response and relaxing the accompanying bronchospasm. Nevertheless, the underlying root problem, oxidative stress, remains unaddressed.

I have read several clinical trials in which patients with asthma showed significantly depleted antioxidants in the extracellular fluid lining of their lungs. Antioxidants vitamin C, vitamin E, and beta-carotene were found at low levels even when the children were not having an acute attack. They also exhibited markedly higher levels of by-products produced by oxidative stress leading to chronic inflammation and hyperactivity of the airways.[2]

Adam's Story

Adam developed a serious case of bronchial asthma at the age of three. It was difficult for his parents to see him struggle simply to breathe. The little boy consequently took several different medications and used a nebulizer (a breathing machine that mixes medication with normal saline) to receive his

Albuterol treatments. But he didn't tolerate his medication well. Because it has a stimulant quality, Adam had a difficult time falling asleep and he struggled with heart palpitations. More discouraging was the fact that even with the medication he was unable to run, play ball, or participate in even the simplest activities. He was frequently fighting colds and made lots of trips to the ER when he had trouble breathing.

The most frightening time came on Adam's fourth birthday. He had developed a cold and quickly became very ill. He began to run a 105-degree temperature, and an x-ray in the ER revealed a severe case of pneumonia and out-of-control asthma. Few of us think of our children possibly dying from pneumonia these days, but the threatening reality certainly crossed the minds of Adam's parents. The birthday boy was fortunate and survived this serious illness, but it left him even weaker and his underlying asthma remained a severe problem.

Adam continued to have problems tolerating the medication the doctors prescribed, though they were doing everything medically possible for him. Their answer wasn't good enough. His father began to look into any other possible therapies that might help his son. As his dad told me Adam's story, he remembered that it had been early summer when they decided to experiment with a potent chewable multivitamin to see if it might help. He distinctly recalls in that early summer Adam would stay near the edge of the swimming pool, barely venturing out into the water. But by the end of that summer, his son was swimming the full length of the pool. Within sixty days Adam changed from a child who could virtually do nothing physically to one who could keep pace with other children. Adam also started playing baseball and eventually even soccer. In fact he qualified for a traveling soccer team over the following four years.

Adam was not only able to play, but he excelled in the sport. (As a physician, I must say soccer is probably the most difficult sport for an asthmatic to play.) He was able to discontinue most of his meds and needed his inhaler only occasionally. Adam is now thirteen years old and continues to be very active in sports. He has chosen to play baseball over soccer and enjoys a life neither he nor his parents ever thought possible.

This young athlete continues to take a potent multivitamin and has added a little grape-seed extract and extra vitamin C to his supplement program. It must be amazing for parents to see their child go from being basically disabled to being normally active. And they certainly don't miss the emergency room visits! How simple and yet profound is the potential life-changing effect of nutritional supplementation.

Asthma and Nutrition

I realize now that when a child comes into my office with severe allergic asthma or hay fever, he has significantly depleted immune and antioxidant defense systems. By the time he visits me, he's been fighting chronic inflammation in his nasal passageways and lungs for some time. In turn it seems these children become allergic to just about everything. They have dark circles under their eyes, they're fatigued, and they take a lot of medication.

I start them on a potent antioxidant and mineral supplement and also add some essential fatty acids in the form of cold-pressed flaxseed oil or sometimes fish oil. As we discussed in Chapter 10, essential fats are important in the body's production of natural anti-inflammatory products, which helps to bring inflammation back under control.

Grape-seed extract is not only a great antioxidant, but it seems to have anti-allergen effects also. This is a strong additional supplement for the child with asthma. I usually recommend that parents give their child 1–2 mg of grape-seed extract per pound of the child's weight. I also give these children additional calcium and magnesium supplements. Magnesium helps relax the bronchospasms of the muscles in the lungs. Since spasms of these muscles is what narrows their airways, this will help open them up.

I always tell parents that it takes about six months to build up a child's antioxidant and immune systems, so they shouldn't get too anxious. If I see them in the spring, I tell parents their child will be doing much better in the fall. *All* of my child patients with hay fever or asthma have improved using this nutritional supplement program. Some stories are dramatic like Adam's, and some reflect just modest improvement, but they all get good results.

Please note: I never have asthmatic children discontinue their medication, because as I shared before, nutritional supplements are not alternative medicine—they are complementary medicine.

I have enjoyed working with children with severe allergies because they respond so well to nutritional supplementation. I remember a story one mother shared shortly after starting her child on my recommended supplements. Her five-year-old was sledding in the snow. As was the custom, the mom was patiently waiting at the door with the child's inhaler. Her child had not been able to undertake any activity, especially outside in the cold, for more than two years without the aid of her inhaler. How amazed the mother grew as her little girl was able to sled in the snow all morning without once needing her inhaler.

I also remember the time our family got together in Sioux City, Iowa. My daughter and niece began racing during our walk along the Missouri River. As all good uncles do, I goaded the girls on, giving my niece a hard time when my daughter beat her. My niece quickly replied she was just thrilled she *could* run. She had not been able to previously due to exertional asthma. I had forgotten that I'd put her on nutritional supplements a few months earlier.

Adult asthmatics can benefit as well. When my wife was suffering from chronic fatigue and fibromyalgia (see Chapter 1), one of the most troublesome problems she had was severe asthma and hay fever. She could not even go into the barn unless she was wearing one of those huge masks that people use when working with hazardous material. My wife loves her horses, and she would do whatever it took to be around them!

Liz was on about five different medications, including allergy shots, in an attempt to control her asthma and allergies. But as soon as she began her aggressive supplement program, her asthma and hay fever dramatically improved. Once her body began rebuilding its defenses, Liz stopped wearing her mask and she came off all medication. On occasion, she still has some allergy problems and will take some of her medication; however, this now occurs only two or three times a year.

Needless to say, our children and many adults are literally under attack from our environment. It is wearing them down, and they need the support of nutritional supplementation. As in the cases of Christian and Adam, medicine does not hold all the answers, and when people are at the end of their rope, they begin to look for other options. But remember, I am not suggesting alternative medicine; I *am* strongly recommending the complementary medicine of nutritional supplements.

The question is, why am I alone in this? Why are physicians so reluctant to recommend that their patients with asthma and allergies take nutritional supplements? It's a mystery to me.

Air Pollution and Chronic Obstructive Pulmonary Disease

There is nothing harder than watching patients, young or old, struggle with every breath, often requiring nasal oxygen twenty-four hours a day. This is the case in those with chronic obstructive pulmonary disease (COPD), which includes emphysema, chronic bronchitis, and bronchiolitis. These patients are hardly able to exert themselves at all and find that their pulmonary disability greatly hampers their joy in living.

Not everyone is able to make a conscious choice to live in a healthy environment, but prevention weighs heavily on my mind. Here again I realize it is not the years in life that are important, but the quality of life we have in those years. We need to do whatever we can now to boost our health or restimulate it if it's weakened.

Air pollution is a key player. Considerable evidence shows that the inhalation of cigarette smoke and airborne pollutants causes the increased oxidative stress that is the underlying cause of COPD.[3] The resultant chronic inflammation in one's airways creates even more oxidative stress, which leads to the damage of sensitive lung tissue. This eventually decreases lung function by disrupting the easy transfer of oxygen through these damaged membranes to the blood.

Studies Show Oxidative Stress is the Cause of COPD

W. MacNee reported in the medical journal *Chest* and at the Novartis Foundation Symposium that he felt that there was considerable scientific evidence that oxidative stress was the cause of COPD. He discovered that many of these patients had depleted antioxidants in their lung tissue due to the increase in oxidative stress and possible dietary deficiency of antioxidants. He stated that antioxidants that have good "bio-availability" (are easily used in the lung) may therefore be potential therapies that would not only protect against the direct injurious effects of oxidants, but also may favorably alter the events that have a central role in the development of COPD.[4]

The progression of COPD is relatively resistant to traditional medical treatment, especially the use of steroids. Obviously, the first task of the physician is usually to help smoking patients to quit. This is not an easy task. I find that it is more difficult to get my patients off of cigarettes than alcohol and even some narcotic medications. Still, the benefit to the patient is tremendous. *Consequently, I will try almost anything to help my patients to quit smoking.*

(A principle you will find throughout this book is that you absolutely must do everything you can to decrease your exposure to those things that create increased oxidative stress. Health is not simply a matter of building up your body's antioxidant defense system.)

If you are developing COPD and have never been a smoker or are not presently smoking, nutritional supplementation may become the best way to slow down the progression of COPD. The basic principles apply with all of these chronic lung diseases just as it does with asthma: the earlier you start an aggressive supplement program, the better your chances of hindering its progression. Once the lung has become seriously damaged, as many smokers have discovered, there is very little chance of significantly improving their lung function.

Cystic Fibrosis

Cystic fibrosis (CF) is a lethal hereditary disease primarily marked by digestive malabsorption (the body doesn't readily absorb the nutrients from one's diet) as well as chronic pulmonary (lung) infections. The malabsorption syndrome found in cystic fibrosis patients is primarily due to deficiencies in the pancreatic enzymes. In addition the epithelial cells of the lungs' airways also do not function well, leading to increased mucus accumulation and bacterial infections. The damage to the lungs that characterizes this disease is again due to the tremendous oxidative stress that is occurring within the lungs' lining.

Several clinical trials have demonstrated that cystic fibrosis patients are seriously deficient in vitamin E, selenium, beta-carotene, and the important antioxidant glutathione, found both within the epithelial cell and epithelial fluid lining of the lung.[5] This continual inflammatory process depletes essential antioxidants needed to protect the patient's lungs and because of the ongoing malabsorption problem, it is impossible for the patient to replenish nutrients adequately.

Cystic fibrosis is a perfect example of what happens when our natural immune and antioxidant defense systems are not able to function properly. The accumulative oxidative damage to the lung tissue occurs quite rapidly, and the majority of these people die before they reach their adult years.

Recent studies have brought encouraging results; namely, the potential in slowing down the progression of this disease by use of nutritional supplements. By combining pancreatic enzyme supplements with potent antioxidant supplementation in patients with cystic fibrosis, researchers were able to bring vitamin E and beta-carotene levels almost back to normal.[6] Clinical trials also indicate that when patients take important antioxidant nutrients, oxidative stress comes back under control, and the patients' depleted immune systems also improve so they are able to fight chronic infections better.

Such clinical studies provide physicians with a strong rationale for supplementing their patients with cystic fibrosis with potent nutritional supplements and pancreatic enzymes. Supplementation can only help improve a patient's condition and hopefully slow down the progression of his or her disease.

Sharlie's Story

Sharlie is a beautiful young woman. She is vibrant and energetic—the picture of health. You would never guess that every day she is fighting for her life. You see, Sharlie was born with cystic fibrosis. She is now twenty-three years old and is already in an elite class when you consider that only 30 percent of these patients make it to adulthood.[7]

No one realizes this more than Sharlie and her mother, Collette. Sharlie's sister died several years ago following a bilateral lung transplant because she also had cystic fibrosis. The two girls were inseparable. Because they both had this chronic disease, they shared a bond most children never get to experience. In fact watching her sister suffer and die following a lung transplant created a deep desire within Sharlie to do whatever she could to protect her own lungs and help win the fight against their common enemy.

Sharlie was fifteen when her sister, Lexi, died. The grief was a heavy burden to bear, but Sharlie also carried the weight of her own struggles—lungs that functioned at only 35 percent capacity most of the time. Her doctor also wanted to put her on the lung-transplant list.

Against the backdrop of her sister's experience, Sharlie decided against this option and chose instead to try improving her disease with the use of potent antioxidant supplements. Lexi had instilled in her this hope. Sharlie saw Lexi respond well to supplements following her lung transplant. Physicians had thought they would lose Lexi shortly after her surgery, but she was a fighter and with the help of nutrients, she recovered remarkably well.

Although Lexi only lived a few months longer, Sharlie was convinced her best option was to try to build up her own body through supplementation. She began taking a potent antioxidant and mineral supplement along with additional vitamin C, calcium, magnesium, and grape-seed extract. She experienced astounding results. Several months later her lung function had improved to over 50 percent. Her physicians were amazed.

Sharlie began to participate in physical education and even some minor sports. She always believed that the more active she could be, the better, even though she continued to have infections and had to be hospitalized from time to time to receive intravenous antibiotics. Despite these small setbacks, Sharlie saw her life and activities rise to almost normal levels.

Her decision not to go on the lung-transplant list but instead start an aggressive supplement program was the best decision of her young life. Sharlie became a symbol of hope for many other children with cystic fibrosis as well.

Unfortunately, Sharlie's battle continues. About three years ago she developed acute shortness of breath. This was more difficult than anything else she had experienced. After her doctor evaluated her, he had to inform her mother that one of Sharlie's lungs collapsed and was not working at all, a condition known as *pneumothorax*.

This certainly depressed Sharlie—at first. But determinedly, she overcame this setback and eventually returned to a near-normal life, fully relying on the one damaged lung she has left. She continues her battle for air and victory over infection. Following a bout of pneumonia that brought her breathing capacity down to 15 percent, she again regained her active lifestyle and shocked her doctors. In fact her breathing capacity has returned to 35 percent.

Sharlie's success story is one of undaunted courage and strength supported by the complementary team of the best of medical attention and nutritional supplements available. Sharlie has learned to live one day at a time. This certainly makes every day a precious gift.

I have known Sharlie now for more than seven years, and she has been a pillar of encouragement to me.

● ● ●

Our lungs are probably most vulnerable to the toxic world in which we now find ourselves having to live. While our bodies do have a great natural defense, they still can become overwhelmed. It is imperative that we build up these natural defenses to their optimal level.

The stories I have shared with you in this chapter are dramatic, and they are true. Isn't it amazing how much better patients with asthma, allergies, and cystic fibrosis do when they learn how to support their lungs' natural antioxidant and immune systems with nutritional supplements? Is this the miracle you've been looking for as well?

THIRTEEN | Neurodegenerative Disease

CARL MOHNER TURNED EIGHTY IN AUGUST OF 2001. ART LOVERS around the world celebrated his birthday but especially those in McAllen, Texas.

Carl, who would become a legend, started out as an actor in Salzburg, Austria, in 1941. After the Second World War disrupted his career for a time, Carl returned to film, and in 1951 he starred in *Vagabunden der Liebe*, the first of more than sixty films. Among his most notable is *The Last Bridge*, which won the Golden Palm Award at the 1953 Cannes Film Festival, as did the French production *Rififii* the following year, now considered a classic. American audiences would best remember Carl as Captain Lindeman in *Sink the Bismark* or as Peter the fish cook in *The Kitchen*.

Despite his success in film, Carl's first love was painting.

Textures and depth became as fascinating to him as the characters in a movie, and to Carl, color spoke the words of life's drama. The canvas became the stage upon which the artist displayed his passion.

One day Carl recognized this same passion in the heart of another painter, Wilma Langhamer, who became his wife in 1978. They left Europe for America, the land of opportunity. They dreamed big dreams and moved to the heart of Texas. Life was good and both artists produced an impressive body of work until 1988, when Carl's life was forever changed.

Carl was diagnosed with Parkinson's disease. The illness rose dark on the horizon of his and Wilma's future and threatened to rob them of all they lived for. But for Carl, change has never been synonymous with lack of success. Predictably, speech became increasingly more difficult for Carl and his ability to walk declined dramatically. But color and drama still danced before his eyes, driving him back to the canvas day after day. In spite of an unknown future, Carl would paint as long as he could.

Some days he felt as though he was swimming through quicksand. Carl's body became the largest obstacle of his life. But challenge was nothing new. While recalling his early years, the painter remembered the rigidity (one hallmark of Parkinson's disease) that was present even years prior to his diagnosis. Carl's strength of will simply had to outmaneuver the limits of his body. He pushed on and continued to paint at a torrential pace, producing more than fifteen hundred paintings between 1990 and 1995.

Though traditional medications helped initially, by the mid-nineties the artist was essentially wheelchair-bound, though he never stopped painting. In the summer of 1999, Carl consulted me to see if nutrition could offer any help. Following my recommendations, Carl started a potent antioxidant and mineral tablet along with a high dose of grape-seed extract and Coenzyme Q10.

After about six months Carl noted some recovery in the movement of his tongue, and he was able to get up and walk for short distances. I decided to increase the amount of grape-seed extract. He reported back to me that he was now able to get up and down to walk about twenty times each day. His physical therapy also helped, and his overall strength began to improve. The most exciting thing for Carl was the fact that he was able to continue to paint. When he painted, he could forget about the Parkinson's disease, at least for a while.

Most would look at Parkinson's as an artist's worst enemy because it significantly affects muscle movements. But Carl continues to show his work at some of the nation's most competitive art shows. In September of 2000 he won first place in 2-D Mixed Media at the highly regarded Plaza Art Fair in Kansas City, Missouri. In March of 2001 at the Bayou City Art Festival in Houston, he again received Best of Mixed Media 2-D.

In honor of Carl's eightieth birthday, Vernon Weckbacher, curator of collection with McAllen International Museum, wrote, "Carl, you see the beautiful and thought-provoking in ordinary things, and through your artwork you impart your special insights to those around you."

As a human being I am awed by the beauty Carl communicates through art. As a physician I am amazed by the fact that he is still able to paint at all, let alone communicate through the medium of art and compete at the highest level of his craft.

"People respond strongly to his art," says Carl's wife, Wilma. "This is what he lives for. When he is absorbed in his work, Parkinson's disease ceases to exist for that moment. It's just him and the painting."[1]

Not only is Carl's life a tribute to his character; it speaks of the empowering results of nutritional medicine. The legend of Carl Mohner is still alive today.

Oxidative Stress and the Brain

Have you ever thought about your ability to think? Thinking about thinking—now there's a concept! When you reach back into your memory banks and recall a vivid childhood experience or that special moment with your family, do you ever marvel at how you can remember even some of the smallest details? Stop reading for a moment and take a look out your window. Have you ever considered with amazement your colored, wide-angled, binocular vision? This is all possible only with God's marvelous creation, the brain.

The brain is our most precious organ because without its full function, we humans simply exist, unable to relate to the world around us. My mother died of an aggressive brain tumor that affected her ability to interpret speech and to speak. It was the most frustrating time of my life because she couldn't understand what we were saying. When we told her we loved her, all we got was in return was a blank stare. Her own words were garbled and made no sense at all. Needless to say, protecting my brain has definitely become a priority.

It should come as no surprise to you now that even the brain (central nervous system) and our nerves (peripheral nervous system) are not out of the reach of oxidative stress. This common enemy has been strongly implicated in a variety of diseases that wreak devastating damage on the brain and nerves, known as *neurodegenerative diseases*.[2] Some of these include Alzheimer's dementia, Parkinson's disease, ALS (Lou Gehrig's disease), multiple sclerosis, and Huntington's chorea. In fact there are several reasons why the brain and the nerves are *especially vulnerable* to oxidative stress:

- Relative to its size, the brain experiences an increased rate of oxidative activity, which creates a significant number of free radicals.

- The normal activity which various chemicals create to establish nerve conduction is a major producer of free radicals.

- The brain and nerve tissue contain relatively low levels of antioxidants.

- Millions of *nonreplicable* cells make up the central nervous system. This means that once they are damaged, they are most likely dysfunctional for life.

- The brain and nervous system are easily disrupted. A small amount of damage in a critical area can cause severe problems.

The brain is the most important organ of our body. Our thoughts, emotions, our ability to reason and communicate with the outside world are all in danger if something damages our brain. How can we best defend this most precious asset? It is not just a matter of trying to avoid the devastation of neurodegenerative diseases, but first and foremost, it is a matter of protecting our ability to think and reason.

Aging of the Brain

Oxidative stress is the leading cause of the aging process. Nowhere is evidence for this concept stronger than when it comes to the actual aging of the brain. Several scientific studies have shown oxidative damage to the mitochondria (the furnace of the cell) and to the DNA of the brain cell. This can lead to the malfunction or even the death of these very sensitive brain cells.[3] As I have pointed out, brain cells do not have the ability to regenerate themselves. So as we lose more and more brain cells throughout our lifetime due to this oxidative damage, the brain simply does not function as well as it did when we were younger. In medical terms this leads to what is called *loss of cognition*. In lay terms this is a decrease in our ability to think or reason. Therefore, oxidative damage to our sensitive brain cells is the greatest enemy to the functioning of our brain.

Aging of the brain is essentially the first stage of degeneration of these very important cells in our body. Just as we don't contract other degenerative diseases out of the blue, people don't just wake up one day and have Alzheimer's dementia or Parkinson's disease. These diseases represent the end stages of oxidative damage to the brain. They are merely part of a progression that begins with the aging of the brain. When eventually enough brain cells are damaged, a disease manifests.

When a patient is first diagnosed as having Parkinson's disease, more than 80 percent of the brain cells in a particular part of the brain called the *substantia nigra* have already been destroyed. The same is true for someone who develops Alzheimer's dementia. These neurodegenerative diseases have actually been developing over a period of ten to twenty years.[4]

Let's look at some of these diseases individually.

Alzheimer's Dementia

Alzheimer's dementia affects more than 2 million Americans and is the major cause for admission to nursing homes.[5] Alzheimer patients not only don't know what day it is, they don't even recognize their own families.

Nothing is more devastating than losing the ability to think. Anyone who has had to deal with Alzheimer's dementia within his family understands just how tragic this is. If you have a loved one who suffers from Alzheimer's, you appreciate the fact that it is the quality of life, not the quantity of life, with which most of us are concerned.

I have treated hundreds of Alzheimer's patients over my career. I have seen them live ten to fifteen years of their lives isolated mentally from their family and friends. As I am writing this chapter, former President Ronald Reagan "celebrated" his ninety-first birthday. Sadly, the news media reported that he has not made a public speech in more than ten years. The passage of another birthday becomes an empty and painful event for those suffering from Alzheimer's dementia and their families.

Numerous studies have presented evidence that clearly demonstrate free radical damage as the cause of Alzheimer's dementia. Recent findings by researchers at Case Western Reserve University concluded that increasing oxidative stress with age most likely accounts for all aspects of Alzheimer's disease. Strong evidence exists that patients with Alzheimer's have significantly depleted levels of antioxidants in their brains as well as high levels of oxidative stress.[6]

There is now great interest in the therapeutic benefits that Alzheimer's patients could receive from antioxidants. The *New England Journal of Medicine* reported in April 1997 a study showing that high doses of vitamin E could significantly decrease the progression of Alzheimer's dementia. Patients with moderate Alzheimer's who took 2,000 IU of vitamin E in supplementation were able to remain at home an additional two to three years longer than the control group members, who took a placebo.[7]

It is not hard to realize the cost savings (not to mention the peace of mind) each family could enjoy by postponing nursing-home care for any length of time. Other clinical trials in which patients with Alzheimer's dementia used various antioxidants such as vitamin C, vitamin A, vitamin E, zinc, selenium, and rutin (a bioflavanoid antioxidant) have also been encouraging.

Parkinson's Disease

A stooped posture, slow voluntary movement, rigidity, and a "pill-rolling" tremor that causes the hands to move back and forth in a "rolling" action characterize Parkinson's disease. Public appearances by Muhammad Ali have made us all more aware of the effects of this debilitating disease. These encumbrances are the reason Carl's story is so profound. Unbelievably, Carl's disease is much more severe than Ali's, and yet he is still able to paint.

A wide variety of studies support the role of free radicals as the underlying cause of Parkinson's.[8] The actual cell death (approximately 80 percent) in the area of the brain called the *substantia nigra* leads to decreased production of dopamine, a substance that allows the brain to function normally.

Studies indicate that patients with early Parkinson's disease who received high doses of vitamin C and vitamin E were able to slow the progression of their disease. They actually avoided taking any medication for their disease for approximately two years longer than the control group. Glutathione and N-acetyl-L-cysteine (both antioxidants) were also effective in protecting the nerves in the substantia nigra from further damage by oxidative stress.[9]

Multiple Sclerosis

Multiple sclerosis affects about 250,000 Americans and is about twice as common in women as in men.[10] Unlike Alzheimer's dementia and Parkinson's disease, in which the brain cells are actually damaged, this disorder affects the myelin sheath (the insulation around the nerve). This breakdown of the myelin, called *demyelination*, results in impairment of the function of the nerve. It is like an electrical wire that shorts out because of a breakdown in the insulation around the wire, and it is responsible for the clinical symptoms of multiple sclerosis.

Dr. S. M. LeVine proposed in 1992 that the hydroxyl free radical found in excess within the myelin sheath caused multiple sclerosis.[11] Other investigators have documented the fact that oxidative stress was significantly higher in patients with MS during a flare-up when compared to MS patients who were stable.[12]

MS differs from the other neurodegenerative diseases in that the mechanism of injury to the central nervous system and peripheral nerves is the immune system, rather than outside toxins. When one's own immune system attacks the myelin sheath, this creates oxidative stress that then damages the nerve.

Multiple sclerosis responds amazingly well to cellular nutrition. There is no doubt in my mind that unlike Alzheimer's dementia and Parkinson's disease, in which irreversible damage has been done to brain cells, the body *does* have the potential to repair damage to the myelin sheath. Placing MS patients on potent antioxidants is critical.

In an attempt to slow or even reverse Parkinson's disease, multiple sclerosis, or Alzheimer's dementia, we haven't yet used antioxidants to their full potential. This is true for a couple of major reasons. First, as I said earlier, by the time a physician is able to diagnose Alzheimer's dementia or Parkinson's disease, a significant number of cells in the brain have already been destroyed. We just don't start treatment soon enough. Second, if we are going to see any success in decreased risk or delayed progression of neurodegenerative diseases, we must research the effects of *antioxidants that cross over into the brain easily*. Third, for patients with a disease like multiple sclerosis, we need to be also using antioxidants that are going to be more effective in getting into both the brain and the nerves. Researchers are not yet studying antioxidants that can smoothly pass through what is known as the *blood brain barrier*.

The Blood Brain Barrier

The brain needs a barrier that separates it from the blood to permit complex nerve signaling. The blood brain barrier is a thick lining of epithelial cells that are present in the small arteries that course through the brain. This lining is designed with very tight junctions, which makes crossover of nutrients into the brain cells particularly difficult.

Important nutrients needed by the brain actually have specialized transporting proteins available allowing them to cross this barrier. At the same time toxic substances, infectious organisms, *and most other nutrients* have difficulty passing through this barrier. This keeps the brain isolated with only its most essential nutrients able to enter. Much like a medieval castle surrounded by water and a high wall whose entry is a drawbridge, so our brain also has significant protection from the dangers of the outside world. God created this amazing defensive barrier for the protection of this very sensitive area of our body.

So you wonder, *What has gone wrong in the case of aging of the brain and neurological disease?*

The neurology department at the Rabin Medical Center in Tel Aviv concluded that as a result of today's environment, the brain is exposed to a significantly increased amount of toxins, such as heavy metals, and thus oxidative stress. The antioxidant defense system is no longer completely effective in protecting this vital organ. They believe that additional antioxidants, which particularly need to be taken in supplementation, have the potential for diminishing or maybe even preventing the damage increased oxidative stress causes. They warn, however, that the antioxidants must be ones that can readily cross over the blood brain barrier.[13]

Let's take a look at each of the important antioxidants needed to protect the sensitive cells in our brain and how well they traverse the blood brain barrier.

The Right Antioxidants for the Brain

Vitamin E

Vitamin E is a fat-soluble antioxidant, which is very important in the protection of brain and peripheral nerve cells. Vitamin E is able to cross through the blood brain barrier, but it does have some difficulty. Researchers have to use very high doses of vitamin E in supplementation in order to increase the level of vitamin E in this area of the body. Therefore, vitamin E is an important antioxidant in protecting brain cells but probably not the best one in this situation.

Vitamin C

Vitamin C can concentrate in the tissue and fluid around the brain and nerves. It is able to pass through the blood brain barrier, and in fact, vitamin C levels are ten times higher in this tissue than in the plasma.[14] When you realize that vitamin C is not only a great antioxidant but also has the ability to regenerate vitamin E and glutathione, it becomes a very important nutrient in protecting brain and nerve cells.

Dr. M. C. Morris reported a study showing that vitamin C and vitamin E given in supplementation to normal patients over the age of sixty-five actually decreased their risk of developing Alzheimer's dementia. This was a small study and larger, more aggressive studies need to be done.[15]

Glutathione

Glutathione is the most important antioxidant within the brain and nerve cells. But this nutrient is difficult to absorb from oral supplements, and its ability to cross the blood brain barrier is not yet clear. Some studies using IV glutathione have shown significant improvements in patients with Parkinson's disease; however, these studies involved only a few patients.[16] The best strategy at this time is to supplement the nutrients the body needs to make its own glutathione (N-acetyl-L-cysteine, niacin, selenium, and vitamin B2). You also need to have those antioxidant nutrients available that regenerate the glutathione so it can be used again and again (vitamin C, alpha-lipoic acid, and CoQ10).

Alpha-Lipoic acid

The medical community is recognizing alpha-lipoic acid more and more as an important antioxidant.[17] It is not only both fat- and water-soluble, it also has the ability to readily cross over the blood brain barrier. It can regenerate vitamin C, vitamin E, intracellular glutathione, and CoQ10.

Another important aspect of alpha-lipoic acid is that it can attach itself to toxic metals in the brain and help eliminate them from the body. Heavy metals such as mercury, aluminum, cadmium, and lead have been implicated in increasing the risk of developing neurodegenerative diseases. These metals tend to deposit themselves in brain tissue because of the high amount of fat concentrated in that part of the body.[18] These metals can cause a significant increased amount of oxidative stress and are extremely difficult to remove from the central nervous system once they are there. Antioxidants that not only are potent but have the ability to help remove these toxic heavy metals will become increasingly important in the prevention and treatment of these diseases.

As a side note, I believe it is wise to eliminate the use of products, such as deodorants and cooking utensils, that contain aluminum. When you realize that heavy metals actually increase the amount of oxidative stress in the body, especially the brain, you will want to decrease your exposure to them.

I anticipate that over the next several years we will hear more and more about mercury toxicity and how it too can cause significant damage to the brain. I would encourage everyone, but especially those with children, to avoid getting mercury amalgam fillings in their teeth. If you ask your dentist about possible alternatives to these mercury amalgams, he does have much safer options. (Don't run out and have all of your mercury fillings removed, though. If it is not done properly, it may cause more harm than if you just leave them alone.)

Coenzyme Q10

Coenzyme Q10, as you will recall, is a very potent antioxidant as well as one of the most important nutrients for the production of energy within the cell. Clinical studies have shown that oxidative damage in the mitochondria (this is where CoQ10 works) is an important aspect in the development of neurodegenerative diseases.[19]

As we age, the level of CoQ10 in our brains and nerve cells decreases significantly. CoQ10 may be a missing link in the prevention of diseases like Alzheimer's dementia and Parkinson's disease; however, further human clinical studies are still necessary. How well CoQ10 passes through the blood brain barrier has not yet been fully evaluated.

Grape-Seed Extract

Studies show that grape-seed extract crosses the blood brain barrier quite readily. It is an exceptionally potent antioxidant, and the mere fact that high concentrations can be obtained in the fluid and cells of the brain and nerve tissue makes it an ideal antioxidant for the brain. My experience shows that this nutrient is a major player in the amazing results I have seen among patients who are suffering from neurodegenerative diseases. I believe it is by far the most important optimizer in these diseases. It is obviously one of the antioxidants that researchers should use further in studies involving these diseases.

Protecting Our Most Precious Asset

Everyone desires to maintain and protect the ability to reason and to think. In fact losing this ability is probably the number-one fear of most of my patients. When a person forgets where he put his keys or can't remember his neighbor's name, he often comes to my office fearing he has developed Alzheimer's dementia.

As we age, we will all have this concern at one time or other. I do not have a fear of dying because of my faith in Christ: to be absent from the body is to be present with the Lord.[20] But after practicing medicine over three decades and seeing so many disabled patients, I do live with a nagging concern of being trapped in my body. I have patients with Alzheimer's dementia who have not recognized their spouses or kids for more than a decade, and yet their general physical health is still good. Walk through a nursing home and you will understand why I am so concerned.

The principle of optimizing our own natural antioxidant defense system is paramount when it comes to protecting the cells in our brain against our common enemy, oxidative stress. Remember, we must focus on *prevention* and *protection*, because once a brain cell is destroyed it is not readily replaced.

There are two main concepts to keep in mind if we are going to have any effect on decreasing the incidence of these seriously disabling diseases: First, we must use a cocktail of antioxidants that will work in synergy while readily crossing over the blood brain barrier. Second, we need to avoid any excessive exposure to the heavy metals I mentioned and other toxins in our environment. Balance is the key, and we must work on decreasing our toxic exposures as well as building up our body's natural defenses.

I believe the cellular nutrition program that I present in Chapter 17 will help the individual who is healthy accomplish his goals for brain health and preservation. If you are already concerned about a decline in your ability to remember things or have a strong history of Alzheimer's in your family, you may want to add some additional nutrients that I call *optimizers*. These are those antioxidants that are known to cross over this blood brain barrier readily, such as grape-seed extract. See Chapter 17 for more details, or, if you are especially concerned, consult me at my website, *www.nutritional-medicine.net*.

Ross's Story

Ross is a cowboy who seems to have walked right off the screen of an old Western. His love of horses goes hand in glove with his love for the sport of roping. And he's good. Western competitors cringe when they see Ross ride into the arena—they know he's stiff competition.

For years Ross was one of the best. He cleaned house at the South Dakota "jackpots." But a few years ago, Ross began noting numbness in his legs. At first he was not too concerned, but then the numbness spread up to his hips and eventually his lower back. The cowboy finally made an appointment with his doctor and after many, many tests, he received the diagnosis of multiple sclerosis.

Ross was devastated. I don't know if cowboys cry, but they can sure be a stubborn lot. This roper wasn't about to give up. He would literally get on his horse, unable to feel the bottom half of his body, and participate in team rop- ing events. Ross now admits it probably wasn't the smartest thing he's ever done, since his balance in the saddle was significantly compromised, but he had to keep living and roping was his life.

It was about this time that Ross began looking into additional therapies for his MS. He heard me speak at a local meeting, and soon after began the nutri- tional supplement program I recommend to my patients with MS. Within months he began to feel better. The numbness and weakness in his legs began to improve.

Today, about three years later, Ross believes that he has fully recovered. The strength in his legs is back to normal, and he has absolutely no numbness in his legs, feet, or lower back. He is back to roping and again feels safe in the saddle. No doubt his fellow roping competitors are back to cringing when Ross pulls up to the rodeo grounds.

●　　●　　●

I have witnessed a number of near-miraculous recoveries from multiple sclerosis. I have personally been involved with several MS patients who have gone from being wheelchair-bound to walking, and I've had several other MS patients who have stabilized their disease with the use of nutritional supplements.

Granted, MS is more than a neurodegenerative disease; it is also an autoim- mune disease that doctors have been able to treat by enhancing the immune system. In fact physicians are now using Betaserone and Avonex (which is actually interferon), drugs known to help improve the immune response. Nutritional supplementation with potent antioxidants, minerals, CoQ10, grape-seed extract, and essential fats do basically the same thing; however, they don't have all the adverse side effects. Again, I always encourage patients to continue taking all their prescription medications along with their supple- ments. Some MS patients do improve so much that they discuss going off their medication with their physicians.

It is quite obvious that the proper functioning of our brain and our nerves is an essential aspect of our health, and we now realize that the main enemy to this central part of our body is oxidative stress. Since brain and nerve cells have a very difficult time regenerating themselves, it is paramount that we protect these sensitive cells from being damaged in the first place.

It will take years of study to prove beyond a shadow of a doubt that supplementing our diet with potent antioxidants that readily cross over the blood brain barrier can effectively protect us against these horrible diseases. But I believe the evidence available in the medical literature is strong enough now to advise my patients to supplement a healthy diet with antioxidants at optimal levels. Such a regimen can only help!

FOURTEEN | Diabetes

WARNING! DO NOT SKIP THIS CHAPTER—EVEN IF YOU HAVE NEVER *been diagnosed with diabetes.*

Diabetes mellitus has become one of the most widespread diseases in existence. Over the past thirty-five years, the industrialized world has seen the number of diabetes cases increase fivefold. In the United States alone, an estimated $150 billion is spent annually on treating diabetes and related complications. An estimated 16 million people in America have diabetes, *but the amazing fact is that approximately half of these individuals don't even know they are diabetic.* This is why even "nondiabetics" must read this chapter.[1]

Even though diabetes itself is a big enough health problem, the side effects of the disease are equally ominous. For example, one-third of the new cases of end-stage kidney disease are due to diabetes. Four out of five diabetic patients eventually will die—not from diabetes itself, but from cardiovascular disease (heart attack, stroke, or peripheral vascular disease) initiated by the diabetes. Did you know that diabetes is the leading cause of amputations and one of the leading causes of blindness in the elderly?[2]

Diabetes mellitus has reached epidemic proportions. With more than 90 percent of these cases known as *type-2 diabetes* (formerly known as *adult-onset diabetes*), we must seriously consider what is going wrong! Type-1 diabetes used to be called juvenile diabetes. This type of diabetes usually occurs in children and is the result of an autoimmune attack on the pancreas. This leaves these children without any insulin; therefore, they must take insulin to survive. However, I am going to focus my attention in this chapter to type-2 diabetes mellitus because this is the type of diabetes that is increasing to epidemic proportions. Why has such an increase in the number of people developing this disease occurred? Is there any way you can personally decrease the risk of developing diabetes?

Absolutely.

Meet Joe

Joe was forty-one when he came into my office for a routine annual physical. He was feeling great and had absolutely no complaints. He just felt he needed a thorough checkup because he hadn't had a physical for several years. During the routine appointment, we drew some blood.

Because Joe felt so good, I was surprised and concerned when my lab technician showed me Joe's blood. It looked pink instead of red. After the technician spun the blood in the centrifuge, the upper portion of the sample looked like cream (meaning it was loaded with fat). The lab report indicated that Joe's cholesterol was 250, his HDL cholesterol was 31, and his triglyceride level was abnormally high at 1,208.

Triglyceride levels should be less than 150 and the triglyceride/HDL ratio should be less than 2. Joe's ratio was nearly 40! Although his fasting blood sugar level was normal, it was soon obvious that Joe had developed Syndrome X—a precursor to diabetes mellitus.

Syndrome X: Is It Killing You?

Like Joe, most people have never heard of Syndrome X, but they certainly need to. Dr. Gerald Reavens, a physician and professor at Stanford University, chose the term to describe a constellation of problems that have a common cause: insulin resistance. Through medical research, Dr. Reavens estimates that more than 80 million adult Americans have Syndrome X.[3]

Let's take a moment to look at the common cause of Syndrome X, the body's developed resistance against insulin.

What Is Insulin Resistance?

Americans are infatuated with a high-carbohydrate, low-fat diet, although in truth, most Americans eat a high-carbohydrate and *high*-fat diet. Over the years our diet has taken its toll, and many of us have become less and less sensitive to our own insulin as a result. Insulin is basically a storage hormone that drives sugar into the cell to be utilized or stored as fat. The body desires to control our blood sugars. Therefore, when the body becomes less sensitive to its own insulin, it compensates by making more insulin. In other words our bodies respond to increasing blood sugar levels by forcing the beta cells of the pancreas to produce more insulin in order to control our blood sugars.

Individuals with insulin resistance need more and more insulin as the years go by to keep their blood sugars normal. Although these elevated insulin levels (hyperinsulinemia) are effective in controlling our blood sugars, they also may lead to some serious health problems. Below is a list of harmful effects elevated insulin levels cause. These are the problems that constitute what Dr. Gerald Reavens has labeled Syndrome X:

- significant inflammation of the arteries, which can cause heart attack and stroke

- elevated blood pressure (hypertension)

- elevated triglycerides—the other fat in the blood beside cholesterol

- lowered HDL (good) cholesterol

- increased LDL (bad) cholesterol

- increased tendency to form blood clots

- development of significant "uncontrolled" weight gain—usually around the middle (called *central obesity*)

When all of the Syndrome X factors are combined, our risk of developing heart disease actually jumps *twentyfold*.[4] Considering the fact the heart disease is the number-one killer in the industrialized world today, we cannot afford to disregard a growing risk of developing it!

After patients have had Syndrome X for several years (maybe even ten to twenty), the beta cells of the pancreas simply wear out and can no longer produce such high levels of insulin. At this point insulin levels begin to drop and blood sugars begin to rise.

At first only mild elevations of blood sugar may develop, which is known as *glucose intolerance* (or *preclinical diabetes*). More than 24 million people in the United States are at this stage of glucose intolerance.[5] Then, usually within a year or two, if no change in lifestyle occurs, full-blown diabetes mellitus will develop. The aging of the arteries then accelerates even faster as blood sugars begin to steadily rise.

What Is the Cause of Insulin Resistance?

Several theories suggest reasons why we become less and less sensitive to our insulin over the years. But I truly believe insulin resistance is the result of the Western diet. Though we focus heavily on cutting back on fats, our love affair with carbohydrates continues. What many Americans don't fully realize is that carbohydrates are simply long chains of sugar that the body absorbs at various rates. Did you know white bread, white flour, pasta, rice, and potatoes release their sugars into the bloodstream even faster than table sugar? It's true. This is why such foods are called *high-glycemic*.

On the other hand foods such as green beans, brussels sprouts, tomatoes, apples, and oranges release their sugars into the bloodstream much more slowly and are therefore considered *low-glycemic* foods.

Our nation tends to eat far too many high-glycemic foods, which in turn causes blood sugars to rise very rapidly and stimulates the release of insulin. When our blood sugar drops, we feel hungry. So we grab a snack or eat a big meal, and the whole process starts all over again. After a period of time, the release of insulin has been overstimulated so often that our bodies simply become less and less sensitive to it. In order for the body to control the blood sugar levels, the pancreas needs to put out higher levels of insulin. It is these elevated levels of insulin that cause the destructive metabolic changes associated with Syndrome X.

How Do You Know If You Have Syndrome X?

Most physicians do not routinely request blood insulin levels for their patients. But there is a simple (although indirect) way to see if you may be developing Syndrome X or insulin resistance. When your blood is tested you will routinely get a lipid profile, which includes the levels of total cholesterol, HDL (good) cholesterol, the LDL (bad) cholesterol, and triglycerides (the other fat in the blood). Most everyone is familiar with the ratio you obtain by dividing the total cholesterol by the HDL cholesterol. But if you divide the triglyceride level by the HDL cholesterol, the ratio you get is an indication of whether you are developing the syndrome. If this ratio is greater than two, you may be starting to develop Syndrome X. Also, if you notice that your blood pressure or that your waistline is increasing, it is even more likely that you are developing a serious case of Syndrome X.

Here's an example of how to do this simple test. Let's say your triglyceride level is 210 and your HDL cholesterol level is 30. Dividing 210 by 30 equals a ratio of 7. Since this is definitely greater than a ratio of 2, you would conclude you have early signs of insulin resistance or Syndrome X.

As soon as a person begins developing insulin resistance, his physician should recommend and support lifestyle changes, because, as I pointed out earlier, this is when cardiovascular damage really begins. Therefore, physicians need to be readily aware of the early signs of developing insulin resistance via the triglycerides/HDL cholesterol ratio. Insulin resistance is totally reversible at this point. We must never be content to wait until a person becomes fully diabetic before treating him.

When a patient treats his insulin resistance with simple but effective lifestyle changes, not only does he prevent accelerated damage to the arteries, but he also avoids diabetes itself. This is true preventive medicine. A healthier lifestyle, not the drugs we prescribe, will make the difference.

Without question, I believe that doctors have overdepended on medication to treat diabetes. Most physicians would agree that diet and exercise can help patients with diabetes, but we simply do not invest enough time in helping them understand that changing those very habits is the *best* offense against the devastating complications of the disease.

I realize it is much easier to write a prescription than to educate and motivate patients to make key changes in exercise and nutrition. But diabetes would be so much better controlled if we did not depend so heavily on meds. Even the representatives of the drug companies who visit my office agree that a high-fiber diet that includes low-glycemic foods is very effective. But they always maintain that patients usually will not make such changes in their diet and therefore must have medication.

This is not what I see. In my practice the majority of patients would rather make lifestyle changes than take more medication, though much depends on the doctor's attitude and approach. Consistently, when I take the time to explain all of this to patients and then ask them what they would like to do, more than 90 percent respond that they would rather try lifestyle adaptations first.

Joe can show us how this works.

How Joe Whipped Syndrome X

Joe was very concerned about his lab results and so felt motivated to immediately change his lifestyle. We placed him on a modest exercise program, a low-glycemic diet, and a regimen of antioxidant and mineral supplementation. I repeated Joe's blood work twelve weeks later and documented amazing improvement: his cholesterol level dropped from 250 to 150, his HDL cholesterol increased 10 points to 41, and his triglyceride level plummeted from 1,208 to 102. His triglyceride/HDL ratio had decreased from 40 to 2.5. Joe accomplished all of this without any medication and within just twelve weeks. Both he and I were thrilled.

If you are in a health predicament like Joe's, you can achieve a similar outcome with the same commitment to lifestyle and eating adjustments. Syndrome X and its deadly ramifications can be beat.

Now let's turn our attention to the progressed development of diabetes and how to reverse its devastating effect on our bodies.

Diagnosis and Monitoring of Diabetes Mellitus

The most common screening technique for diabetes is a fasting blood sugar test like the one I gave Joe. Physicians also use a sugar-challenge test, in which an individual is given a sugar load (a pop-like drink that is loaded with sugar), and then takes a blood sugar level test two hours later.

Most physicians believe that a two-hour blood sugar above 190 (definitely above 200) is the level needed to diagnose diabetes. A normal two-hour blood sugar level should be less than 110 and definitely less than 130. (Patients who have a slightly elevated fasting blood sugar and a two-hour blood sugar between 130 and 190 are classified as having glucose intolerance—preclinical diabetes—and not actual diabetes.)

Since a blood sugar measurement indicates only how a patient is doing at a particular moment, another helpful test is a hemoglobin A1C, which reveals the amount of sugar found in a red blood cell. (I like to have a patient with diabetes or diabetic tendencies have this test done every four to six months.) Since our red blood cells remain in the body for approximately 140 days, this test is a great indicator of how well a patient is truly controlling his or her diabetes. The normal range for a hemoglobin A1C in most labs is 3.5 to 5.7.

The goal for a diabetic is to keep tight control so that the hemoglobin A1C remains below 6.5 percent. When patients are able to do this, their risk of developing a secondary complication is less than 3 percent. But if they maintain a hemoglobin A1C of greater than 9 percent, their risk of developing a secondary complication related to diabetes jumps to 60 percent. This comes as a shock, especially in light of the fact that the average *treated* diabetic in the United States maintains a hemoglobin A1C of 9.2. Needless to say, this is not a great endorsement for our health-care system when it comes to diabetes.

Of greater concern is the fact that at the time of actual diagnosis of diabetes by a physician, a majority (more than 60 percent) of these patients already have major cardiovascular disease.[6] This puts the patient at a disadvantage before he even starts treatment. You see, once insulin resistance begins, the process of atherosclerosis (hardening of the arteries) accelerates dramatically. This is why it is critical for physicians to recognize Syndrome X in their patients as soon as possible and encourage lifestyle changes that can correct the problem. A patient may have Syndrome X many years before he truly becomes diabetic. By this time treatment to reverse damage is simply too late.

Obesity

All of us have heard the media and physicians claim that the reason diabetes is becoming epidemic in the United States and the industrialized world is because so many people are developing obesity. This is really not the case. The media has put the cart before the horse, so to speak. Insulin resistance (Syndrome X) leads to *central* obesity, not the other way around. In fact obesity is a major aspect of this syndrome.

What do I mean by *central obesity?* This has to do with how your weight is distributed in your body. If it is evenly dispersed all over or you are heavy in the bottom (pear-shaped), you may need to drop some weight, but in relation to Syndrome X, you are fine. But if you have gained substantial weight around your waistline (are apple-shaped), you may be in trouble.

I have had many patients in their late twenties or early thirties come into my office complaining that they are gaining a significant amount of weight. What bothers them is the fact that their eating habits and activity level have not changed, but they've put on thirty to forty pounds in the past two or three years. Why are they gaining so much? Typically it is because the patient has developed a resistance to insulin. These patients have begun various diet programs but were not able to lose much weight. Such diets are essentially high-carbohydrate, low-fat; this makes the insulin resistance only worse. If these people do not correct the underlying problem for their weight gain—insulin resistance—they will not lose weight. How frustrating it must be to keep going back to their support group but never coming close to losing the kind of weight the others are!

I encourage all of my patients to begin balancing their diet by eating low-glycemic carbohydrates with *good protein* and *good fat* (which I'll explain later in this chapter). When this diet is combined with a modest exercise program and cellular nutrition (Chapter 17), the underlying insulin resistance may be corrected. The weight will then start coming off as mysteriously as it came on. My patients are often amazed at how they are losing weight without really even trying. They feel good, and their energy level is remarkable.

Please know that when I say *diet,* I'm not referring to a fad diet. A fad diet is something that you start with the intention of someday quitting (the sooner, the better!). Instead, I'm talking about a healthy lifestyle that has the side effect of fat loss. I work aggressively with my patients for about twelve weeks so they know exactly how to apply these principles to the way they like to eat. Losing weight is not the answer. Correcting insulin resistance is the key.

Treating Diabetes

All physicians agree that we should first give our patients a chance to improve their diabetes by encouraging them to make effective lifestyle changes. But as I've noted, many physicians simply give lip service to such changes while relying heavily on medications to control the disease.

If we are going to make any significant headway in decreasing the number of diabetics, as well as help current diabetics improve control of their disease, two things have to happen. First, we need to pay more attention to insulin resistance, the underlying problem in the overwhelming majority of cases of type 2 diabetes mellitus, and not simply focus on treating blood sugar levels (see box). Second, we need to aggressively encourage lifestyle changes that will improve insulin sensitivity. I strongly believe that in type 2 diabetes mellitus, physicians should rely on medication as a last resort.

Doctors Are Treating the Wrong Thing

In a review article for the Mayo Clinic, Dr. James O'Keefe stated: "Therapeutic efforts in patients with diabetes have focused predominantly on normalizing increased blood sugar levels while often ignoring many of these other modifiable risks, which are caused by the underlying insulin resistance."[7]

This accounts, in part, for the fact that 80 percent of diabetics still die of cardiovascular disease.[8] I maintain that treatment of the underlying cause of most diabetes, insulin resistance, is a much better way to confront and control diabetes.

Lifestyle Changes Spelled Out

What many people don't realize is how *simple* the lifestyle changes are for treating the primary underlying problem in both diabetes mellitus and insulin resistance. We are talking about modest exercise, eating in such a manner as not to spike the blood sugar, and taking some basic nutritional supplements to improve the patient's sensitivity to his or her own insulin. When you combine all three of these changes, as you saw in Joe's case, the results are phenomenal.

Let's look at each of these ingredients in a healthy response to insulin resistance.

Diet

In my opinion too many doctors make major mistakes in the diet they recommend to their diabetic patients. Since the greatest risk for these patients is cardiovascular disease, the American Diabetic Association has remained primarily concerned about the amount of fat in people's diets. Therefore, the diet the ADA and many dieticians support is a high-carbohydrate, low-fat diet.

Diabetics have religiously followed the ADA's recommendations for the past thirty-five years. In the mid-seventies, 80 percent of diabetics were dying from cardiovascular disease. And as we enter the new millennium, 80 percent of diabetics are still dying from cardiovascular disease.[9] Shouldn't this warrant some reconsideration of our approach?

Once we understand that we need to treat the underlying resistance to insulin, we recognize that carbohydrates are the main concern. This is contrary to dietitians who believe that "a carbohydrate is a carbohydrate" and that the source does not matter. This thinking completely ignores the glycemic index (the rate at which the body absorbs various carbohydrates and turns them into simple sugar).

Numerous studies demonstrate that some carbohydrates release their sugars more rapidly than others.[10] The more complex carbohydrates (ones with a lot of fiber) like beans, cauliflower, brussels sprouts, and apples release their sugars slowly. When these low-glycemic carbohydrates are combined with good proteins and good fats in a balanced meal, the blood sugar does not spike. This is critical in controlling diabetes. If the blood sugar doesn't rise significantly after a meal—a major factor in diabetic control—there is no problem of having to bring it back down with drugs.

Dr. Walter C. Willett, chief of nutrition and preventive medicine at Harvard Medical School, proposed in his book *Eat, Drink, and Be Healthy* that we must rethink the food pyramid the USDA recommends. The bottom rung should be low-glycemic carbohydrates, while high-glycemic foods (white bread, white flour, pasta, rice, and potatoes) belong at the top of the food pyramid with all the sweets.[11]

Everyone realizes how bad sweets are for diabetics. But few realize that high-glycemic foods raise blood sugar much faster than eating candy does. When I finally convince my diabetic patients to eat low-glycemic carbohydrates combined with good protein and good fat, their diabetic control improves dramatically, and their bodies become more sensitive to their own insulin.

Basic Diet Instruction

The following are *good* fats, proteins, and carbohydrates. When you combine these in each meal or snack you eat, your blood sugar will not jump to dangerous levels that need controlling.

The best protein and fats come from vegetables and vegetable oils. Avocados, olive oil, nuts, beans, soy, and so on are great sources of protein and contain fats that will actually lower your cholesterol.

The best carbohydrates come from fresh whole fruits and vegetables. Avoid all processed foods. An apple is better than apple juice. Whole grains are essential, and avoiding processed grains is critical in developing a healthy diet for everyone, especially the diabetic.

The next best protein and fats come from fish. Cold-water fish such as mackerel, tuna, salmon, and sardines contain those fats we discussed in Chapter 10: omega-3 fatty acids. These fats not only lower cholesterol levels but also decrease the overall inflammation in our bodies.

The next best protein comes from fowl, because the fat of the bird is on the outside and not marbled into the meat. Even though this is saturated fat, by removing the skin from the meat you still can have a very lean protein meal.

Obviously the worst fats and protein come from our red meats and dairy products. If you are going to eat red meat, at least eat the leanest cut you can. You should avoid dairy products except for low-fat cottage cheese, milk, and egg whites. If you are going to eat eggs, try to get range-fed chicken eggs, which contain omega-3 fatty acids.

Some of the worst fats that you can eat are the *trans-fatty acids*. These are called *rancid fats* because they are so harmful to our bodies. Get used to looking at labels and any time you see "partially hydrogenated" anything—don't buy it.

These are the basic diet instructions I share with my diabetics and my patients who have developed Syndrome X, like Joe. The focus of this book does not allow me to get into the fine details of the diet I recommend to my patients. For those curious about diets and Syndrome X, I recommend a couple of books: *40-30-30 Fat Burning Nutrition* by Gene and Joyce Daoust, and *A Week in the Zone* by Barry Sears. These straightforward books recommend the 40-30-30 balance: 40% carbohydrates, 30% protein, and 30% fat—this is the balance of these macronutrients recommended during a meal. I tend to use more of a 50-25-25 ratio in my office, but the principles are the same.

This is not a high-protein meal program like the Adkin's diet. This is a healthy diet you can continue the rest of your life. If everyone would eat this way, exercise, and take some basic micronutrients, the diabetic epidemic would be nonexistent.

When you eat this way, instead of stimulating the release of insulin, you stimulate the release of the opposite hormone called *glucagon*. Glucagon utilizes fat, lowers blood pressure, decreases triglycerides and LDL cholesterol, and raises HDL cholesterol. This is eating for hormonal control rather than calorie control. I tell my patients that they are eating a healthy diet that has the side effect of fat loss.

Exercise

Modest exercise has tremendous health benefits. And exercise is especially critical for the patient with Syndrome X or diabetes mellitus. Why? Studies show that exercise makes patients significantly more sensitive to their own insulin and is, therefore, a critical part of the lifestyle change needed for diabetics and those who have insulin resistance.

The exercise program should include a balance of aerobic and weight-resistance exercise done at least three, and not more than five or six, times per week. It is important that people get involved in an exercise program that they enjoy. No one has to become a marathon runner. Even a thirty- to forty-minute brisk walk three times weekly makes a tremendous difference.

Nutritional Supplements

Several clinical trials have found that individuals with preclinical diabetes or impaired glucose tolerance have significantly increased levels of oxidative stress. Often these same people have depleted antioxidant defense systems. Other studies have revealed that oxidative stress was more significant in those with secondary complications of diabetes, such as retinopathy (damage caused by diabetes to the blood vessels in the back of the eye that can lead to blindness) or cardiovascular disease. The researchers conducting these studies concluded that antioxidant supplements should be added to the traditional diabetic treatments as a way to help reduce these complications.[12]

Several studies have shown that all antioxidants may improve insulin resistance. It is important that a diabetic take a good mixture of several antioxidants in supplementation at optimal—not RDA—levels (see Chapter 17). In my research and medical practice, I have learned that several micronutrients are normally deficient in patients with preclinical and full-blown diabetes:

Chromium is critical in the metabolism of glucose and the action of insulin, but studies show that 90 percent of the American population has a chromium deficiency. Chromium has been shown to greatly improve insulin sensitivity, especially in those who are deficient in this mineral.[13] Diabetic patients and patients with Syndrome X need 300 mcg of chromium in supplementation.

Vitamin E not only improves antioxidant defenses but also seems to help the body in the problem of insulin resistance. Research reveals that a low vitamin E level is an independent and strong predictor for the development of adult-onset diabetes. Individuals who have low levels of vitamin E have a fivefold higher risk of developing diabetes than those with a normal amount of vitamin E.

Magnesium deficit has been associated with both type 1 and type 2 diabetes, as well as an increased risk of retinopathy in diabetic patients. Studies show that when this deficiency is corrected in the elderly, insulin function improves significantly.[14]

Unfortunately, diagnosing magnesium deficiency is very difficult. Typically, serum magnesium levels are tested where only a trace amount of the body's total magnesium is located. Cellular levels of magnesium are much more sensitive and accurate; however, these can be tested only in research labs, not in hospitals. This is why magnesium deficiency is so underdiagnosed.

We all need at least 400–500 mg of magnesium in supplementation.

Vanadium is not a well-known mineral, but it is very important for the diabetic. It has been show to significantly increase insulin sensitivity when taken in supplementation. A diabetic needs to take 50–100 mcg of vanadium in supplementation each day.

I have been amazed at what can be achieved with patients who are willing to change their diet, start exercising, and take nutritional supplements with key minerals and antioxidants that improve the body's sensitivity to insulin. Along those lines, here's one case history I love to tell.

Matt's Story

Matt, whose longtime dream had been to join the Peace Corps, came to me for the organization's required physical. During the exam, Matt complained that he had been really thirsty and urinating quite often. Since he was only twenty-three, he did not understand why he needed to go to the bathroom several times each night.

I drew a blood sugar blood test for Matt, and it came back at 590, a level so dangerously high I admitted him to the hospital and started immediate infusion of intravenous insulin. When his blood sugar did not respond well to this treatment, I consulted an endocrinologist. This physician also had problems controlling Matt's diabetes and ended up giving him higher doses of insulin than he had ever given a patient before. At one point Matt was taking ninety units of insulin twice a day (a normal dose is approximately ten).

After Matt finally stabilized and left the hospital, I suggested that he make lifestyle changes while still taking insulin. He agreed and began working out, eating food that would not spike his blood sugars, and taking mineral and antioxidant tablets. Matt was dedicated and did well staying with his program. His weight started to fall and gradually he was able to decrease the amounts of prescribed insulin. Month after month he improved.

Four months after his visit for the physical, Matt came into my office and informed me that his blood sugars were normal and that he wasn't taking any insulin. Knowing his history, I really didn't believe him. So I checked his fasting blood sugar. The result was 84. I then challenged him with a sugar load and checked his blood sugar two hours later. It was 88—within normal limits. His hemoglobin A1C was 5.4, which also was normal. Matt was no longer diabetic.

I then had the difficult task of writing a letter to the Peace Corps, explaining that Matt was at one time an insulin-dependent diabetic but now was no longer even diabetic. I feared that the unusual report might disqualify Matt and end his dream of service. But the Peace Corps repeated his blood work and concluded too that he was no longer diabetic.

Matt joined the Peace Corps and spent two years in Africa. The organization actually flew him out of the bush to a hospital every six months for tests to be sure his blood sugars remained normal. He said staying with the balanced diet I had recommended was a challenge, but by eating the unprocessed grains that were available, he did very well.

I had the privilege of seeing Matt again last month in my office. He is now finished with his tour in the Peace Corps and still maintains normal blood sugars. He also informed me that he stayed with the program I initially laid out for him, and he has dropped his weight from 315 pounds down to 205 pounds. He said the weight just came off without his even trying, once his blood sugars returned to normal and he had corrected the insulin resistance.

• • •

I believe that many other persons who are borderline or fully diabetic can experience a similar change in their physical health. If you struggle with diabetes, are you willing to invest in necessary lifestyle changes to free yourself from a decreased dependency on medication and live a healthier life? Remember, you want to control your diabetes and at least maintain a hemoglobin A1C of less than 6.5. This is very difficult to do with medication alone. Applying these principles to your own life will significantly improve your diabetic control. You should watch your blood sugars closely when you begin these lifestyle adjustments; if the blood sugars drop too much, you need to consult your doctor so he can adjust your medication.

As I said earlier, diabetes mellitus is increasing at epidemic proportions. In spite of the billions of dollars spent on this disease, we are losing the battle. Physicians and laypeople alike must refocus their attitudes and attack insulin resistance rather than elevated blood sugars. When we see elevated triglyceride levels along with lower HDL cholesterol levels, hypertension, or unusual weight gain, we need to recognize the possible development of Syndrome X and accelerated cardiovascular damage that may have already begun.

Rather than simply treating the diseases that insulin resistance causes, we need to aggressively treat the insulin resistance itself. Isn't it amazing that such simple lifestyle changes can effect a near-miracle: the disappearance of diabetes?

FIFTEEN | Chronic Fatigue and Fibromyalgia

"I'M JUST SO TIRED—ALL THE TIME. IT IS DIFFICULT FOR ME TO concentrate. I can't remember the last time I felt good. In fact, I'm having a hard time remembering a lot of things. I know something is wrong with me. I don't have any energy, and I seem to catch every bug that comes along. I need help, but I don't know where to start. Maybe it's my thyroid—my family has a history of thyroid problems."

Have you ever uttered these statements? I can't tell you the number of patients who consult my web page seeking help or come into my office with these kinds of complaints. They are frustrated and discouraged with their ongoing condition. In the thirty years I've been in private practice, I'd have to say that these are some of the most common ailments I hear about.

During a consult visit, doctors usually ask, "Do you hurt anywhere? Do you have any other symptoms?" Then we run through a complete review of potential complaints, trying to find out if the patient is suffering from symptoms ranging from headaches to chest discomfort to diarrhea. Often patients answer in the negative to all of the specific questions and sigh, "I am just really tired and have absolutely no energy."

When physicians confront this situation, they usually recommend a complete physical exam with a comprehensive chemistry profile. On the next visit the physician will go over the patient's complaints again and review past, present, and family health histories. He will conduct another physical exam, and after the evaluation is complete the doctor will carefully review the laboratory data. Occasionally he discovers evidence of hypothyroidism, diabetes, anemia, or some other disease process that is causing these symptoms of fatigue. But the overwhelming majority of the time, he finds nothing that sufficiently explains why the patient is feeling so tired and worn out.

At this point most physicians begin questioning the patient about possible signs of increased stress or symptoms of depression. If this line of questioning doesn't reveal any apparent explanation, tension begins to fill the air. The patient starts to realize the doctor is not finding anything wrong. And the doctor may even insinuate that the problem is all in the patient's head. Of course, this is not a verbal exchange, but the unspoken reality is most certainly communicated through abrupt tones and body language. (If you have ever been in a situation like this, you understand fully what I'm talking about.)

What just happened? Physicians want to help their patients, and most often they feel the only way to accomplish this task is by finding a disease process and beginning treatment with a prescription. When they can't find anything wrong or can't write a prescription, doctors become uncomfortable with the mounting pressure to provide an explanation and course of action to make the patient feel better. A doctor may dismiss the visit by standing up and saying, "Well, you are really in excellent health—I can't find anything that would explain your symptoms. Just give it some time and see if you feel better."

If you have experienced something similar, you know you've nothing else to do but turn and leave the doctor's office, frustrated. You're certain you had already given it "plenty of time" before you went to see the doctor in the first place! Beyond doubt, you're not well, and now that the doctor can't find anything wrong, even you begin to wonder if it's truly all psychosomatic.

But the frustration is only beginning. You may determine to follow your physician's advice and give yourself more time while trying to do everything in your power to take better care of yourself. Instead of getting better, though, you either don't improve or even get worse. Where do you go from there? Do you get a second opinion? If you do see another medical doctor, chances are good that he will not find anything wrong either. Anxiety and disappointment with the health-care system begin to peak.

On the one hand you are happy that no one has found anything serious; but on the other, you're angry because no one has answers. In fact you begin to feel like an annoyance and are intimidated about going back. This is when a close friend or family member tells you about an alternative health-care practitioner who was really able to help him with the same problem.

Alternative Health Care

Your journey continues as you turn from the medical community in search of a solution. You decide to seek out a more natural route, alternative health care, because traditional medicine has been no help (to the contrary, it probably made you feel worse!). To your surprise, the alternative health-care provider identifies a problem right away. He may claim that you have "systemic yeast," "leaky gut syndrome," or "subclinical hypothyroidism" as the cause of your symptoms.

Alternative practitioners typically do a hair or eye analysis, blood work, urine test, or muscle exam to determine exactly what you need. Then they usually recommend certain herbs, bowel cleanses, diet changes, and nutritional supplementation to correct the diagnosed problem.

Relief and hope mounts because someone is *finally listening* and can actually provide an explanation for the exhaustion, even if the diagnosis is not entirely correct. Even though your health and your sense of well-being may improve because of lifestyle changes, you may begin to realize you should be feeling better and are still "not yourself." Here's why. Alternative-care practitioners focus on trying to find out exactly which nutritional deficiencies you may have and then try to correct them. But they are not correcting the underlying problem, which is oxidative stress. Most likely, you will remain frustrated, having to continue reading and doing anything you can to find help.

Immunologically Depressed

Have you ever been "sick and tired of being sick and tired"? Many people with fatigue leave their doctors' offices with a prescription for antidepressants. When the physician is not able to find anything wrong, he assumes that the patient is depressed. But I have learned that when patients do not feel well and do not have the energy to perform their duties, they get discouraged and start second-guessing themselves. They wonder if they will ever have the energy to be high-spirited again. As time wears on, they do get down—they become depressed. But this is truly different from a depression you see in a patient who is emotionally depressed. This is why I label these patients "immunologically depressed."

The increased oxidative stress people experience not only creates fatigue but also depletes the immune system. When patients use nutritional supplements to bring oxidative stress back under control, they not only feel better, but they begin to function normally again, which makes them feel better still. I always enjoy it when my patients tell me during a return visit, "I am not depressed anymore. Can I go off of the antidepressants the other doctor prescribed? They never really helped me anyway."

The very serious illnesses in this book that I have discussed are merely the end result of prolonged exposure to excessive oxidative stress within the body. People do not realize that lasting fatigue is on the same continuum as severe illness. Though many will not develop a serious illness initially, when their bodies are under the attack of prolonged oxidative stress, they will continue to wear down until a serious disease develops.

If I were to do a study of people passing by on the sidewalk to determine how many don't feel up to par (have significant amounts of residual fatigue), my guess is that the numbers would be shocking. Let me tell you what I have learned over the past seven years of practicing nutritional medicine.

You don't just wake up one morning with chronic fatigue syndrome or fibromyalgia. My patients who are coming in not feeling well, complaining of fatigue, frequent infections, poor sleep, anxiety, and depression are also suffering from the beginning stages of degeneration due to increased oxidative stress. I can almost tell by looking at a person's face if he is under excessive oxidative stress. His face is drawn and ash-colored, and he does not look vibrant or healthy. If we don't address the underlying problem effectively, these patients will most likely develop chronic fatigue, fibromyalgia, or even more serious degenerative diseases.

I no longer send my weary patients out the door with the comment, "I can't find anything wrong with you." I know this causes immunological depression and may lead to more serious conditions. I now encourage people to look at their lifestyles and environments for possible clues of increased stress or toxic exposures. They need to attempt to eliminate causes of increased oxidative stress (see Chapter 3) as much as is humanly possible. It is important for them to think about their lifestyles and their stress levels. Are they being exposed to excessive toxins like secondary cigarette smoke, herbicides, pesticides, and airborne pollutants? I encourage them to get proper rest, start to exercise regularly, and begin to eat a healthy diet. I then start them on a potent antioxidant tablet, mineral tablet, and some grape-seed extract and have them return to see me in the clinic in about four to six weeks.

Unlike alternative practitioners, I look for the root cause of the symptoms.

I don't need to do the expensive testing they do (most has been shown to be inaccurate anyway) because I am not trying to correct any one particular nutritional deficiency—but rather the underlying threat of oxidative stress. Instead, I attempt to provide the cell with *all* of the micronutrients at optimal levels. The cell will decide what it does and does not need.

Consistent with the medical literature, I've found that bringing oxidative stress back under control with cellular nutrition is by far the most effective means of redeeming one's health. With this approach the overwhelming majority of my patients are able to return to a normal life.

Follow-up is also very important. It is simply amazing to see how many patients return feeling almost normal again. Their improvement is often dramatic, obvious in their face and skin tone. And to think for years I used to just send these patients out the door with no hope and no counsel! The right treatment was there all along.

A Story of Chronic Fatigue and Fibromyalgia

Judie's experience with fibromyalgia began in November of 1990. She had been a person who was seldom sick, but that year she became very ill with flulike symptoms that caused her body to ache so severely that she thought at any moment she would have to be rushed to the emergency room. It took almost two weeks before she recovered fully from this virus.

She spent one spring day in 1991 outdoors doing yard work. This was not an unusual task for her, but when she awoke the next morning, she felt as if she had moved furniture for three days. She thought she had probably just overdone it the day before. Little did she realize that this was only the beginning.

The next problem she encountered was a sleep disorder. Although she tried a number of solutions, such as medication, less coffee, and warm milk, nothing seemed to help. She continued to struggle with erratic sleep patterns for the next *four* years. She also experienced confusion, memory loss, and visual disturbances. Soon she became aware of joint pain, knots in her shoulders, headaches, and a sore throat—those symptoms were more apparent in the morning hours; but the sore throat and mild headaches were a constant problem. She realized something very serious was affecting the quality of her health.

When she began waking each morning with stiffness, she knew it was time to seek medical help. At this point she was getting only three to four hours of sleep at night, and those few hours were not restful. Her nerves were frayed, and every little noise and action set her off.

The medication I gave her enabled her sleeping pattern to change somewhat, but after using the medication for a year she started to develop side effects. This particular medication made her heart race and caused extreme mood swings and horrible nightmares. She was convinced the medication was doing more harm than good, so she decided to stop taking it.

It was time for Judie to have a checkup with me. She told me later that she dreaded having to tell me she had thrown away the medicine I'd prescribed and had decided to try vitamin therapy instead. I'd always told her that if people ate properly they could get all the nutrients the body needs. To her surprise, I had recently become more open-minded concerning the effects of antioxidants in the healing process. I even placed her on an aggressive nutritional supplement program.

In September of 1995 Judie started this program of nutritional supplements. The effects were amazing! Within three weeks she noticed a significant energy surge. No longer did she have to go to bed at 8:30 P.M. in order to make it through the next day. And shortly after feeling more energy, she became aware that the painful knots in her shoulder blades had disappeared. By November the joint and muscle aches started to subside. In December she had minor surgery, and some of the symptoms returned shortly afterward. But she increased her antioxidant intake, and within two weeks the symptoms were no longer a problem.

In March of 1996 she slept her first eight-hour night. She was delighted to notice her sleep pattern was once again one of normal, deep sleep. Her nerves were no longer frayed, and she felt a pervasive sense of wellness returning. Confusion cleared, and her thinking process began to improve. Six years later, she is still doing well.

The Root Cause

Chronic fatigue and fibromyalgia are both devastating and disabling diseases that the medical community believes to be different expressions of the same disease. Chronic fatigue patients have severe fatigue but more sore throats, swollen glands, and fever; fibromyalgia patients suffer from severe fatigue and total body pain. As I've said, I believe they share a common cause—oxidative stress.

No specific treatment exists for either of these diseases. As a result, fibromyalgia used to be called *psychosomatic rheumatism.* In fact, many physicians still believe this disease is just in the patient's head. No doubt these are frustrating illnesses for both the physician and the patient. Unfortunately, traditional medicine offers only symptomatic medications: nonsteroidal anti-inflammatories, muscle relaxants, antidepressants, and sleeping medication. Physicians also refer the patient to a support group and tell them they just need to learn to live with it.

Let's look at these illnesses in more detail and see what better treatments are available.

Fibromyalgia/Chronic Fatigue

Nearly 8 million patients in the U.S. alone may be suffering from fibromyalgia—and eight out of nine are women. You may wonder: Does personality play a role in who might be prone to the disease? Perhaps. Statistics seem to indicate these women are perfectionists who are especially sensitive.

These patients are most often living in total pain, are extremely fatigued, and suffer from lack of sleep. They wake up stiff, experience mental confusion, and many have irritable bowel and TMJ syndrome, which is when an individual develops a very painful jaw along with headaches.

Most fibromyalgia patients come into my office toting a stack of medical records from several different doctors, because a diagnosis of fibromyalgia usually takes an average of seven to eight years to get! Talk about frustration! They have been tested from top to bottom with absolutely no abnormal findings. The only way to truly discern whether a patient has fibromyalgia is to do specific tender-point testing of eighteen predetermined areas. If eleven or more of these areas are significantly tender when only mild pressure is applied, the patient is diagnosed with fibromyalgia.

A majority develop fibromyalgia following a serious illness, a major injury (especially of the neck), or a substantially stressful time in their lives. As you have learned, all of these situations greatly increase the amount of free radicals our bodies produce. Once this disease starts, there seems to be no letting up. One may have an occasional good day but have little or no reserve. And after doing too much in any given day, including exercising, one may become too stressed or ill, and severe fatigue will set in for the next two to three weeks.

Treatment: Capturing the Disease

Once I have made the diagnosis of fibromyalgia or chronic fatigue syndrome, I focus on bringing oxidative stress back under control. I can accomplish this best, of course, through cellular nutrition, which I detail in Chapter 17. I also strongly encourage a healthy diet as well as a low-impact exercise program. I always caution against exercising two days in a row and recommend combining a mild aerobic exercise program with a light-weight-resistance program.

Remember, this is a chronic, lifelong disease, so rebuilding one's health takes time. It is always exciting when a person responds quickly and dramatically, but this is not the typical scenario. I always encourage my patients to commit at least six months to improving their condition. They may not necessarily be where they want to be in that time, but they know that they are on the right track.

Once my patients begin to see improvement, it is like the lights have just been turned on. Typically skeptical at first, they become excited when there is no doubt that their health is improving. I call this "capturing" the disease—they are actually bringing oxidative stress back under control.

The first victory a patient notices is the fact that she is no longer experiencing "mental fog." It becomes easier to think and concentrate on the task at hand. Next, sleep patterns improve. She can actually get a more restful sleep and see a significant increase in energy. The last thing that usually improves is the pain. That is correct: *the pain finally begins to subside.*

By following this protocol my fibromyalgia patients have had good-to-excellent results about 70 to 75 percent of the time. Several hundred people suffering from fibromyalgia over the past seven years have improved dramatically following my nutritional program I've detailed specifically on my web page located at *www.nutritional-medicine.net.*

I believe that when a patient fails to respond well, it is because we cannot bring her oxidative stress under control via oral supplementation alone. This is when I recommend that my patients go to a medical center specializing in IV nutritional supplementation. IV therapy is necessary for them to "capture" their disease and finally begin to improve. Oral therapy then helps manage their condition.

Now keep in mind, these people still have fibromyalgia or chronic fatigue. I am not presenting a cure. Instead, I am empowering patients to control their disease rather than having the illness control them. Over the years, I have watched as so many gradually got better, increasing their reserve. It does take time, but their hope and determination are well rewarded.

Mariano's Story

Mariano introduced himself to me in Philadelphia where I had been speaking. He had driven two hundred miles, hoping for a chance to talk to me. He shared his story with me that day, and it touched my heart.

Mariano had suffered with such severe fibromyalgia that he consumed more than three hundred Advil tablets a month to control the pain. He had to leave his office, where he had a psychiatric practice, by 3:30 each day and was in bed by or before 7:00 P.M. because of overwhelming fatigue.

It was at this point he started the nutritional program I have used with all of my fibromyalgia patients. Within a few weeks Mariano began noticing a substantial difference. He became more alert, and his fatigue began to lessen. He was able to work a full day, and he was going to bed later and later. He then began to note improvement in his pain. After a month or so, his pain improved so remarkably he didn't need the Advil at all.

Mariano got his life back. He is again able to maintain a full psychiatric practice and has added four to five hours back to each of his days. It has now been several years since I first met Mariano, and he continues to do well. Since his practice often involves treating the mental problems of patients who are suffering from chronic degenerative diseases, he certainly has a thorough understanding of how these diseases can affect a person's life.

●   ●   ●

The growing shift to alternative health care should serve as a wake-up call to the medical community. People are becoming more and more frustrated with the health-care system that their medical insurance covers. So they are frequently resorting to self-help methods and alternative care for answers, even though they have to foot the bill. Simply put, people are sick and tired of being sick and tired. In spite of the fact that physicians are prescribing antidepressants at record levels, alternative care is flourishing in the United States and around the world.

Why? Perhaps patients seek alternative care as a result of experiences like the scenario I presented at the beginning of the chapter, but I also believe it has much to do with patients not having the love affair with medication that most physicians believe they do. Patients want options other than taking more medication.

We physicians must realize that we are primarily responsible for the major shift of medical care to alternative health-care providers. We frustrate our patients into making alternative decisions. After all, the overwhelming majority of patients do see their physicians first. Most physicians now appreciate the benefits of a healthy diet and a modest exercise program. But these same physicians do so without fully appreciating or understanding the consequences of oxidative stress. If they did, they would strongly encourage their patients to start taking high-quality potent nutritional supplements—instead of discouraging them. Not only would tremendous improvements occur in their patients' symptoms, doctors would see a significant decline in patients' seeking alternative health care.

PART III

NUTRITIONAL MEDICINE

SIXTEEN | Physicians' Bias Against Nutritional Supplements

As I REFLECT BACK ON MY FIRST YEARS OF MEDICAL PRACTICE, I clearly remember my own bias against nutritional supplements. So I don't have to look any farther than myself when it comes to understanding the basic prejudice doctors have. I am sure that my past feelings are not too different from those of the majority of physicians practicing medicine today.

I remember telling my patients that they could get everything that they needed from their food, if they would just eat a healthy diet. "You just go down to your local grocery store and buy the right kind of foods, and you don't have to take any of those supplements," I would insist. "Taking vitamins is a waste of money."

If that didn't convince them, I would share a study or two that showed a vitamin to be harmful. I remember that the negative studies were really the only ones on vitamins of which I was really aware. After all, when negative studies were publicized in the lay media or medical journals, I would tell myself, "See, you were right all along about those vitamins. It's a shame that these charlatans have played such scams on my patients."

Part of the reason I have changed my mind about vitamins is the quality of our diet.

The Typical American Diet

I have a confession to make right here, right now: I have actually eaten out in a fast-food restaurant. All right, if you must know the gritty details, I had a

Big Mac, French fries, a large Coke—super-sized, even—and a hot apple pie. But you must also know that that was years ago. I have learned a little something about eating since then.

Did you find yourself chuckling at the thought of a person confessing to something we all have done more often than we want to admit? In spite of the knowledge that fast food is about the worst excuse for fuel we can ingest into our bodies, we line up by the fryer vat, waiting to pay our hard-earned cash for the detriment of our future health. Friends, *knowing* and *doing* are two different realities. As much lip service as we give to losing weight and eating healthy, in reality, it's just not happening.

Approximately 40 percent of our calories in the typical American diet come from fat, and most of this is saturated fat (the bad stuff). The September 1997 issue of the medical journal *Pediatrics* reported that only 1 percent of children in the United States get the proper RDA levels of the essential nutrients from their diets.[1] Not only are children not getting proper nutrition for their growing bodies, they are establishing poor eating habits in childhood that usually persist into their adult years. It has amazed me how many of these young teenagers already have full-blown insulin resistance.

The Second National Health and Nutritional Survey evaluated twelve thousand American adults and their eating habits. Here are some of their findings:

- Seventeen percent of the population did not eat any vegetables.

- Excluding potatoes and salads, 50 percent of the population did not eat any vegetables. In other words only half of the population ate *garden* vegetables.

- Only 41 percent consumed any fruit or fruit juices.

- Only 10 percent of the population met the USDA guideline of eating a minimum of five servings of fruits and vegetables a day. Among African Americans, only 5 percent ate the recommended amounts.[2]

Even though physicians and registered dieticians recommend that we consume multiple servings of fruits and vegetables daily, our society is falling woefully short. This study shows us that if we exclude French fries and baked potatoes, more than half of the population is not eating *any* vegetables.

Worse yet, almost 60 percent of the population is not eating *any* fruits. In truth Americans are not eating a healthy diet even though they know better.

Is it any wonder that more than 50 percent of our nation is now considered to be *significantly* overweight? When you combine these poor eating habits with the high-glycemic foods discussed in Chapter 14, it is no wonder that we have an epidemic of insulin resistance and diabetes in the U.S. If I were to challenge you to go out and not eat any white bread, white flour, pasta, rice, and potatoes for two weeks, you would quickly realize why so many people (more than 80 million Americans) have developed insulin resistance known as Syndrome X.

Quality of Food in the U.S.

No other nation on the face of the earth has produced the abundance of food that America has over the past half century. But when you look at the quality of our food from a health perspective, there are definite concerns. The processes used to produce and preserve our foods today have had a serious effect on the quality of this tremendous food supply. Rex Beach wrote in his report to the U.S. Senate:

> Do you know that most of us today are suffering from certain dangerous diet deficiencies, which cannot be remedied until the depleted soils from which our foods come are brought into proper mineral balance? The alarming fact is that foods—fruits and vegetables and grains—now being raised on millions of acres of land that no longer contain enough of certain minerals, are starving us no matter how much we eat.[3]

Beach made this statement in 1936. And in the almost seventy years since Beach's plea to the Senate, little has been done to improve our nation's depleted soil; in fact, the situation is much worse today than ever before in history.[4] Five major minerals (calcium, magnesium, chloride, phosphorous, and potassium) and at least sixteen trace minerals are essential for optimal health. Plants cannot create minerals. They must absorb them from the soil. And if our soils do not have these minerals, our plants will not have them either.

And they don't. Why? Organic fertilizers that contain these minerals are expensive and difficult to obtain. U.S. farmers manage their costs by using fertilizers that replenish the soil with only nitrogen, phosphorous, and potassium (called NPK). With these NPK fertilizers, farmers are able to grow good-looking grains and produce, though the crops remain depleted in all the other necessary minerals. Unfortunately, economics is the driving force behind American agriculture, causing farmers to be more concerned about bushels per acre than the nutrient content of the food they harvest.

Few would argue about the quality of our foods and its decline compared to foods of a generation or two ago. Hybrid grains, vegetables, and fruits have increased in popularity. These hybrid seeds boast big, luscious products that are more resistant to diseases. The nutrient content of hybrids, however, is significantly less than that of their natural counterparts. The farmer is paid according to bushels per acre—not for the quality of his produce. Agriculture too has become a demanding and politically charged industry. In spite of our need for nutrition, the bottom line for farmers is making a living, and hybrid produce makes it possible.

Our food industry, due to special transportation and storage techniques, has been able to make a wide variety of fruits and vegetables available nationwide throughout the year. The variety is good. But these are made available at a sacrifice. Green harvesting means picking fruits and vegetables before they are mature. Shipping food over long distances requires cold storage and other preservation methods, which allow for depletion of vital nutrients. Our food is also highly processed. For example, the refinement process of our flour to create white bread removes more than twenty-three essential nutrients, magnesium being one of the most important. Our food industry then puts about eight of these nutrients back into our bread and calls it "enriched."

Did you know?

- In the process of making white flour, our removing the germ from the outer portion of the grain costs us more than 80 percent of flour's magnesium.
- The processing of our meats removes 50 to 70 percent of vitamin B6.
- Cold storage removes up to 50 percent of tangerines' vitamin C.
- Asparagus stored for just one week can lose 90 percent of its vitamin C.[5]

It is a fact that our food is significantly deficient in vital nutrients, even at the time we purchase them; however, the way we prepare our foods is perhaps even more critical. Overcooking, delay in preparing fresh foods, and freezing foods are some of the reasons our foods lose nutritional value. For example:

- Fresh salads and cut vegetables and fruits lose more than 40 to 50 percent of their value if they sit for more than three hours.
- Vitamin C is vulnerable to both heat and cold, and prolonged storage depletes it.
- The preparation of food significantly decreases folic acid.
- Freezing meats can destroy more than 50 percent of the B vitamins.[6]

We began with depleted nutrients in our soils, which NPK fertilizers made worse. Then came the hybrid grains that produced nutrient-depleted foods. Modern processing and food storage caused further depletion of the quality of our foods. We then take these foods home and continue to create further depletion because of storage and preparation. These all make good, solid arguments as to why we should be supplementing our diets with high-quality nutritional supplements.

You must understand, however, that these are not the primary reasons I recommend the use of nutritional supplementation. Though these conditions have proven to be detrimental to our American health, our understanding of nutrition has been equally if not more harmful. We must rethink the meaning of RDAs—recommended daily allowances.

Optimal Levels Versus RDA Levels

First, you must understand how recommended daily allowances were developed in the first place. The RDAs started in the early 1920s and 1930s as minimal requirements of ten essential nutrients that could help us avoid acute deficiency diseases. These are diseases like scurvy (deficiency of vitamin C), rickets (deficiency of vitamin D), and pellagra (deficiency of niacin). In other words if you consumed the RDAs for vitamin C, vitamin D, and niacin, you would not develop any of these illnesses.

Admittedly, the recommended daily allowances have done their job. In my three decades of clinical practice, I have never seen one of these diseases. They still occur, but they are rare. In fact the Center for Disease Control does not even track these diseases anymore.

The list of nutrients included in the RDAs grew over the next two decades, and in the early 1950s the definition of RDAs expanded to include the amounts of nutrients needed for normal growth and development.

Despite the fact that RDAs have proved useful, most physicians and laypeople tend to assign more meaning to RDA standards than they should. This is due in part to the U.S. government's requiring that all food and supplement labels give their percentages according to the RDAs. But after spending the past several years learning about nutritional supplementation and its effect on chronic degenerative diseases, I have become convinced of one overriding truth: RDAs have absolutely *nothing* to do with chronic degenerative diseases.

I believe this one simple truth is the cause of more confusion about the health benefits of nutritional supplementation than any other fact. Physicians are trained to believe that the RDAs are the level of nutrients that are needed by the body for optimal health. This false assumption is the main reason I believe physicians, registered dietitians, nutritionists, and the health-care community in general show such resistance to nutritional supplementation.

As you search the medical literature about oxidative stress and the amount of nutrients needed to prevent it, the level of nutritional supplementation is significantly greater than RDA levels. A good example of this is vitamin E. The recommended daily allowance of vitamin E is 10 IU, and in some schedules as high as 30 IU. The average American diet contains 8–10 IU. According to medical literature, you do not begin to see any health benefits until ingesting *100* IU of vitamin E in supplementation. This health benefit seems to improve all the way up to 400 IU and even higher. (Most physicians who understand supplementation would agree that one must consume at least 400 IU of vitamin E daily.)

The RDA for vitamin C is 60 mg, even though discussions over the past few years suggest this needs to be increased to 200 mg daily. The medical literature, on the other hand, indicates that our bodies need at least *1,000 mg* of vitamin C before health benefits result. This benefit improves even more as we reach 2,000 mg.

I could go through all the major nutrients and list the optimal levels shown to provide health benefit in the medical literature. In each case there is no relationship to the RDAs. Again, recommended daily allowances have nothing to do with chronic degenerative diseases. To get an idea of how much food we'd need to consume in order to achieve these optimal levels of nutrients, see Table 1.

Table 1 — Amount of Food Needed to Achieve these Optimal Levels of Nutrients

Vitamin E (450 IU)
- 33 heads of spinach
- 27 pounds of butter
- 80 medium avocados
- 80 mangos
- 2 lbs. of sunflower seeds
- 23 cups of wheat germ
- 1.5 quarts of corn oil

Vitamin D (600 IU)
- 22 large egg yolks
- 6 cups of fortified milk
- 30 tablespoons of margarine
- 15 ounces of shrimp

Vitamin C (1300 mg)
- 17 medium kiwifruit
- 16 medium oranges
- 160 medium apples (including the skin)
- 10.5 cups of fresh orange juice
- 16 cups of raw chopped broccoli

Folate (1 mg)
- 3.8 cups of cooked asparagus
- 4 cups of black beans
- 20 medium oranges
- 10 cups of brussel sprouts
- 3.8 cups of cooked spinach

Vitamin B6 (27 mg)
- 41 medium bananas
- 38 medium baked potatoes with skin
- 77 cups of lentils
- 15 lbs. of chicken breast
- 18 cups of wheat germ

Riboflavin (27 mg)
- 22 ounces of beef liver
- 16 cups of lowfat yogurt
- 9 dozen eggs
- 3.25 gallons of lowfat milk
- 64 cups of cooked spinach

Thiamin (27 mg)
- 135 cups of brown rice
- 2 lbs. of ham
- 3 lbs. of sunflower seeds
- 64 cups of green peas
- 12 cups of wheat germ

There is simply no way to achieve these optimal levels of nutrients through food. If you desire to decrease your risk of developing a chronic degenerative disease, you *must* supplement your diet.

You may be heaving a sigh of relief, thinking, *Oh, good. I'm covered because I take a multivitamin.* Don't relax just yet. Taking a daily multivitamin cannot protect you from degenerative disease either. Multivitamins are primarily based on RDAs. It is rare to see any reference in the medical literature to a health benefit in patients who are simply taking a multivitamin. You must take *significant* amounts of high-quality antioxidants and minerals if you have any desire to prevent or slow down the chronic degenerative diseases described in this book.

The obvious next question should be, Is it safe to take these supplements at these optimal levels? As a physician who was not always convinced that taking supplements was a good idea, I would frequently discuss such dangers with my patients. I'm sure your physician can quote a few studies that showed a harm in taking supplements. Are there dangers? Sure there are. We need to discuss these in detail.

Dangers Versus Safety of Nutritional Supplements

Throughout this book I have related medical evidence that demonstrates the effectiveness of nutritional supplements in preventing and/or slowing the progression of degenerative diseases. For these supplements to be effective for this purpose, we must take them over a lifetime. We'll want to use them at much higher levels than the RDAs, and we're already an unhealthy population, so it is critical these nutrients be virtually free of any toxic effects and safe for use in strong doses.

Antioxidants are certainly safe when taken correctly. Nutritional supplements are simply nutrients we get from our foods, only at a higher level than is possible from regular eating. On the other hand pharmaceutical drugs may possess *some* clinical benefit in preventing *some* chronic diseases, but they inherently create a risk to the patient.

Every time a physician prescribes a medication, especially if it is for the treatment of a chronic illness, he must explain the potential danger for the use of that drug. "The medications we prescribe," said Dr. Bruce Pomeranz in the April 15, 1998 *Journal of the American Medical Association,* "cause over 100,000 deaths a year." He also states that another 2.1 million patients have serious complications because of medications.[7] Nutrients carry no such dangers.

In my next book titled *Death by Prescription* (to be released by Thomas Nelson Publishers in 2003), I explain the inherent dangers of all medication and the pitfalls in determining potential side effects of medication. There you will find a very practical and understandable guideline for avoiding suffering and possibly death from an adverse drug reaction.

Since properly prescribed and administered medication is the fourth leading cause of death in the U.S., it is time physicians and health-care providers begin to face this major health crisis.[8] Medical professionals speak out and fight to decrease the risk of heart disease, stroke, and cancer. But why don't we talk about helping our patients decrease their risk of suffering or dying from the medications we prescribe?

While our profession essentially ignores this significant cause of death, I find it terribly ironic that physicians continue to discourage their patients from taking supplements on the premise that supplements could be dangerous to their health!

Only a handful of deaths have been reported in the last several years related to supplements. And these have been cases in which individuals have taken *many times* the amounts recommended in this book of a particular nutrient such as niacin. Other reports involved accidental overdose of supplements in children.

Nonetheless, we still must be aware of the fact that nutritional supplements can be toxic if taken in very high amounts. Let's take a look at the main toxic effects of individual nutrients.

Vitamin A

Of all the nutritional supplements, straight vitamin A causes the most concern. Vitamin A toxicity can occur in adults who take in excess of 50,000 IU per day for a prolonged period of time. A lower dose may also create toxicity if the patient has liver disease. Signs of vitamin A toxicity include dry skin, brittle nails, hair loss, gingivitis, anorexia, nausea, fatigue, and irritability.

Accidental ingestion of a single large dose of vitamin A by children (100,000–300,000 IU) can cause acute toxicity. This may present as headache, vomiting, and stupor because of the increase in intracranial pressure.[9] A study reported in the January 2, 2002, issue of the *Journal of the American Medical Association* indicates that vitamin A can be harmful for normal bone function, leading to an increase in hip fractures.

Women must avoid vitamin A supplementation during pregnancy. Dosages as low as 5,000–10,000 IU are believed to have caused birth defects.[10]

I never recommend taking straight vitamin A in supplements. We can meet the need for vitamin A within the body by simply taking beta-carotene and the mixed carotenoids. These are very safe, and the body is able to turn beta-carotene into vitamin A as the need arises without any risk of toxicity.

Beta-Carotene

Beta-carotene has been used in high doses over several years without a single reported adverse effect. Some individuals develop a yellowing of the skin called *carotenodermia*, but this is totally benign and reverses completely once the beta-carotene is reduced or discontinued.

Vitamin E

Although vitamin E is a fat-soluble vitamin, it has a fantastic safety record. Clinical trials of vitamin supplementation as high as 3,200 IU per day have not shown any adverse effects. In addition studies have shown that vitamin E inhibits platelet aggregation and decreases the risk of blood clots in much the same way aspirin does. This property of vitamin E is actually a benefit in reducing heart disease. Researchers believe that vitamin E actually improves the effectiveness of aspirin in patients with heart disease.[11]

Vitamin C

Vitamin C is safe even at very high doses, although some people may experience abdominal bloating, gas, or diarrhea. At one point, there was concern that vitamin C supplementation might increase the risk of kidney stones. This was found in only one clinical trial, however, and the last four similar trials did not substantiate this concern.[12]

Vitamin D

Vitamin D has great potential to cause toxicity. Dosages greater than 1,500 IU are not recommended. In most cases I do not recommend supplementing with vitamin D in doses greater than 800 IU per day. Vitamin D toxicity may increase the blood levels of calcium, cause deposits of calcium in internal organs, and increase the risk of kidney stones.[13]

Interestingly, recent studies reported in the *New England Journal of Medicine* have shown that 93 percent of the people in Boston are deficient in vitamin D—even those taking multivitamins.[14] Other studies are now revealing that the RDA of vitamin D is too low (200 IU) and patients need to take 500–800 IU of vitamin D, which is again is an optimal level. This dosage is still considered to be well within a safe range.[15]

Niacin (Vitamin B3)

High doses of niacin supplementation may create flushing to the skin, nausea, and liver damage. Clinical studies have shown slow-released products with niacin may decrease the risk of flushing, but they may also increase the risk of liver damage.[16]

Many people use high doses of niacin as a natural way to decrease their cholesterol levels. Using pharmaceutical levels of niacin supplementation should always be done under the direction of a physician. The levels of niacin recommended in Chapter 17 are in a very safe range. Niacin is now also being used along with the statin drugs, which are especially effective in lowering cholesterol.

Vitamin B6 (Pyridoxine)

Vitamin B6 is one of the few water-soluble vitamins with a possible risk of toxicity. Doses greater than 2,000 mg can cause symptoms of nerve toxicity. But people using doses between 50 and 100 mg daily have not reported any cases of toxicity.[17] Definitely be careful when using higher doses of vitamin B6.

Folic Acid

Folic-acid supplementation may mask an underlying vitamin B12 deficiency. Therefore, people should always take vitamin B12 supplements in tandem with folic acid. However, there has not been reported any serious problems of taking folic acid even up to 5 grams per day. This is another reason that cellular nutrition is a safe way to supplement your diet.

Choline

Choline is generally well tolerated, although at very high doses (20 g per day), it can create a fishy odor and cause some nausea, diarrhea, and abdominal pain.[18]

Calcium

People tolerate doses of calcium supplements of up to 2,000 mg. It was once thought that high levels of calcium supplementation could lead to an increase in kidney stones; however, a recent study showed that higher levels of calcium actually decreased the risk of kidney stones. In other words those patients who had the highest intake of calcium actually had the lowest risk of kidney stones.[19]

Iodine

Iodine supplementation greater than 750 mcg can suppress thyroid hormone secretion. Reports have also been made of acne-like skin eruptions at higher levels of iodine intake.[20]

Iron

Concern about the use of iron—especially inorganic iron—in supplementation has increased. Americans generally get plenty of iron, and supplementation of this nutrient may create an iron overload, which has been associated with increased risk of heart disease in males. There is some concern iron supplementation may actually increase oxidative stress.[21]

Manganese

Manganese taken in supplementation is very safe, although there are reports of people who develop manganese toxicity from their environment. This is usually seen in those who mine manganese or are exposed to high levels in the environment. These individuals may begin to hallucinate and become very irritable.[22]

Molybdenum

Molybdenum is quite safe. A daily intake of greater than 10–15 mcg, however, may lead to goutlike symptoms.[23]

Selenium

Several clinical trials, which used doses in the range of 400–500 mcg daily, have found selenium to be safe.[24] I believe, however, doses of selenium supplementation should be less than 300 mcg daily. Symptoms of selenium toxicity include depression, irritability, nausea, vomiting, and hair loss.[25]

No toxic effects have been associated with supplementation of vitamin K, vitamin B1 (thiamin), vitamin B2 (riboflavin), biotin, vitamin B5 (pantethine), inositol, vitamin B12, chromium, silicon, CoQ10, boron, and alpha-lipoic acid.[26]

A Physician's Defense

I am certain my medical training was not much different from that of the overwhelming majority of physicians practicing medicine today. I essentially received no formal medical training in nutrition. It was not a required class at my medical school. This is not shocking, since, as I mentioned in Chapter 1, a course in nutrition is still *required* in only a few of the medical schools around the country.

Elective courses in nutrition are offered in about 50 percent of the medical schools;[27] however, as I mentioned in the introduction, recent studies have shown that only about 6 percent of the graduating medical students have received any training in nutrition. I would boldly state that even those students who received a course in nutrition did not study much about nutritional supplementation. This simply is not the focus of our medical training. Physicians learn about the diagnosis and treatment of diseases. It wasn't until I spent the last seven years devouring the medical literature on this subject that my opinion changed.

For the first twenty-three years of my practice, I was a typical physician in regard to my knowledge and opinion about nutritional supplements. My opinions about vitamins were strong and filled with emotion, and my patients truly believed me. Maybe that was because I was an M.D., and we are supposed to know everything about health. We don't!

Physicians base their use of medications, and in turn nutritional supplements, on reliable clinical trials reported in the medical literature. And not every study involving nutritional supplements has showed significant benefit. In some cases they've actually shown potential harm. Both the public media and medical literature publicize these negative studies.

As I described in the introduction of this chapter, when I was not a fan of nutritional supplementation, I knew about these negative studies and quoted them frequently to my patients. At that time, one negative study seemed to negate hundreds of good-quality studies that showed supplements' health benefits. Because any individual who reads the medical literature will encounter several of these studies, I feel it is important to address a few of the most publicized ones.

The Case Against Nutritional Supplements

The Finnish Study

This study based in Finland is probably one of the most-quoted when it comes to nutritional supplementation. Nearly thirty thousand heavy smokers participated in this. They were divided into four equal groups.

Group 1 did not receive anything.

Group 2 received dl-alpha-tocopherol (synthetic vitamin E).

Group 3 received synthetic beta-carotene.

Group 4 received both dl-alpha-tocopherol and beta-carotene.

Researchers followed these subjects over a period of five to eight years. Most of these smokers did not quit smoking during the trial. The study showed no reduction in the incidence of lung cancer in any of the groups receiving the supplements. But even more of a concern was the fact that those individuals who were taking the beta-carotene supplementation actually showed an increase in the incidence of lung cancer. This came as a shock to the investigators because several earlier studies had shown a reduced risk in those patients who had high levels of vitamin E and beta carotene in their diets or blood streams.

The CARET Study

This study involved eighteen thousand smokers and asbestos workers who lived in Washington State. These patients received 15 mg of beta-carotene and 25,000 IU of straight vitamin A. Researchers monitored these patients over a four-year span, and again no decrease in the risk of cancer occurred in patients who were taking the supplements. Again, there was actually an increase in the incidence of lung cancer in the group that was taking beta-carotene and vitamin A.[29]

The Physicians' Health Study

This study followed more than twenty-two thousand U.S. healthy male physicians who took either 50 mg of beta-carotene or a placebo every other day for twelve years. The supplementation showed no benefit or negative effect when it came to lung cancer or heart disease.[30]

My Response

Are the findings of these studies unsettling for you? At first glance, they seem disappointing, but let's take a closer look. All of these studies clearly show that if you are a smoker or are at high risk of developing lung cancer, you should not take beta-carotene alone. I often look for principles that become evident in the medical literature. Here is a perfect example: you should not take a single nutrient at very high levels, especially if you are a smoker. Beta-carotene and other antioxidants have the potential to become pro-oxidants in these situations. A pro-oxidant is a nutrient that can actually cause an increase in the number of free radicals you produce.

Rather than discouraging supplement use altogether, these studies indicate that using beta-carotene alone or with just vitamin E with smokers is not wise.

Also, the fact that the Finnish Study used dl-alpha-tocopherol, synthetic vitamin E, concerns me. Other studies have shown this synthetic vitamin E to cause problems rather than reduce them.[31] Instead, most studies reported in the medical literature use d-alpha-tocopherol, which is a natural vitamin E.

I have already shared my concern that most studies are done with just one or two antioxidants, with researchers looking for the "magic bullet." But an understanding of oxidative stress and how it can damage the body forces us to realize that a one- or two-nutrient approach is like trying to bring down a locomotive with a rifle.

We must also consider the known fact that lung cancer takes twenty to thirty years to develop, so in reality the Finnish Study was destined to fail from the beginning. These patients were heavy smokers who were placing their bodies under tremendous oxidative stress. These patients—and all of those in the studies cited—needed *cellular nutrition* (supplementation of complete and balanced antioxidants and minerals at optimal levels), not magic bullets.

A More Recent Study

Another study reported in the November 29, 2001 issue of the *New England Journal of Medicine* has also received fairly heavy media attention. The Simvastatin (Zocor) and Niacin Study involved 160 patients with elevated cholesterol levels and hardening of the arteries who were assigned to one of four groups:

Group 1 was the control group and so received nothing

Group 2 received Zocor and niacin

Group 3 received vitamin E, vitamin C, selenium, and beta-carotene.

Group 4 received Zocor, niacin, vitamin E, vitamin C, selenium, and beta-carotene.

Group 2 did the best and actually showed some minor reversal of the hardening of their arteries. The antioxidant group (Group 3) was the next best with significant improvement. But Group 4, which received a combination of Zocor and antioxidants, did not see as much of a rise in their HDL (good) cholesterol. This finding was a marginal finding and was not statistically significant. Yet the negative press that has come from these marginal findings has led the overwhelming majority of doctors to quickly claim that taking vitamin E with their prescription cholesterol-lowering drugs blocks the beneficial effects of their drugs.

Physicians tend to ignore the hundreds of studies that show significant health benefits of nutritional supplements not only with heart disease but with all of the chronic degenerative diseases. As you have learned throughout this book, heart disease is not a disease of cholesterol but rather an inflammatory disease of the artery. This same study also showed that the LDL cholesterol showed a 35 percent increase in resistance to oxidation in the antioxidant group than in the groups taking the "statin" drugs.

The media did not pick up this finding, nor did they announce it to the whole world. They also do not tell you that patients who are taking statin drugs significantly decrease the CoQ10 levels of the body. Many researchers feel the underlying reason why some of the patients who are taking "statin" drugs develop muscle pain and even muscle destruction is because of these very low CoQ10 levels in the muscle. Physicians will usually base their decision about the health benefits of nutritional supplements on a study such as this. However, they totally ignore the hundreds of studies that show health benefits with the use of nutritional supplements.

•   •   •

I hope and pray that independent-thinking physicians will take a look at the studies I have detailed in this book. I encourage physicians to be open-minded skeptics and examine the benefits they can offer their patients through nutritional supplements. Rather than relying on RDAs or trying to attack oxidative stress with one vitamin at a time, we must learn how cellular nutrition is the best approach to handling the underlying problem of oxidative stress.

Most importantly, we need to keep in mind the overall concept of oxidative stress, and understand the health benefit patients can realize by building up their bodies' *natural* antioxidant defense system. The result is nothing less than lives changed forever, for better.

SEVENTEEN | Cellular Nutrition: Putting It All Together

I HAVE SPOKEN OF SOME OF THE MOST FRUSTRATING OR PAINFUL diseases doctors encounter in their patients, but I must now testify to the deepest fulfillment of a physician: watching men, women, and children of all ages living life at its fullest again after a debilitating disease. These people are back in control of their health, instead of their illnesses controlling them.

But here is the honest truth: I have never seen patients achieve this kind of response with traditional medicine alone. You could look at one or two cases and believe that the results were a "supernatural" miracle of God. But this natural healing ability has been there all along. We have been marvelously and wonderfully made. Medical science is now just showing us that we have to optimize these natural healing systems that are already present. We must take advantage of humanity's most tremendous asset in healing, "the host," which is our own body.

Sometimes the physician has a tough time getting any healing to occur. Nothing frustrates a physician more than dealing with a compromised immune system. This happens frequently with people suffering from full-blown AIDS or those who have been taking chemotherapeutic drugs.

The infections these patients get are severe and sometimes remarkably unusual. Because the patient's own immune system is barely functioning, physicians are left with few options other than to pull out their most potent antibiotics on a wish and a prayer that the patient will respond. In this setting the physician realizes the importance of having an immune system that is working at an optimal level. Our drugs may be great; however, without the help of the body's own healing power, they are really not that effective.

Doctors need both drugs *and* a healthy immune system. Again, this is why I call the use of high-quality, nutritional supplements *complementary medicine.*

Optimal Levels of Nutrition

You must remember, especially if you are a health-care practitioner, that vitamin E, selenium, calcium, magnesium, and vitamin C are simply nutrients that we should be getting from our foods. But we continue to study them as if they were drugs. Drugs must go through rigorous clinical trials to assure they are safe and effective, because they are synthetic substances that disrupt natural enzyme systems in order to create a therapeutic result. In the last chapter I discussed possible safety risks posed by nutritional supplements. But the risks are few, especially compared with drugs. This is because vitamin E, vitamin C, selenium, and so on are actually *natural* substances that support natural enzyme, antioxidant, and immune systems.

Because we now have the means of producing nutritional supplements, we are able to provide these nutrients at optimal levels. Optimal levels are those levels that have been shown to provide a health benefit in the medical literature. These are not RDA levels (see Chapter 16). When these nutrients are combined and taken together in supplementation at these optimal levels, the results are simply amazing.

Cellular nutrition is simply providing all nutrients to the cell at optimal levels. This allows the cell to decide what it really does and does not need. I don't have to worry about determining in which nutrients the cell is deficient. I simply provide all of the important nutrients at optimal levels and let the cells do their work. This approach corrects any nutritional deficiencies over the next few months.

Bakers know the true art of baking bread, but with the handy use of automatic bread machines, just about anyone can give it a try. We don't have to do much anymore in the way of technique. If you dump in all the right ingredients (in the right balance—this is even guaranteed thanks to premixed packets), you get a luscious, warm loaf of fresh homemade bread in about a couple of hours or so. But what if you don't have a little packet of ingredients and you forget the yeast? What if you use too much salt? This is the same approach we use with cellular nutrition. You want to provide all the necessary

Table 1 Basic Nutritional Supplement Recommendations

ANTIOXIDANTS	The more and varied your antioxidants, the better.
VITAMIN A	I do not recommend the use of straight vitamin A because of its potential toxicity. Instead supplement with a mixture of mixed carotenoids. Carotenoids become vitamin A in the body as the body has need and they have no toxicity problems.
CAROTENOIDS	It is important to have a mixture of carotenoids rather than taking only beta-carotene. • Beta-carotene 10,000 to 15,000 IU • Lycopene 1 to 3 mg • Lutein/Zeaxanthin 1 to 6 mg • Alpha carotene 500 to 800 mcg
VITAMIN C	A mixture of vitamin C is important, especially calcium, potassium, zinc, and magnesium ascorbates, which are much more potent in handling oxidative stress. • 1000 to 2000 mg
VITAMIN E	It is important to be getting a mixture of natural vitamin Es: d-alpha tocopherol, d-gamma tocopherol, and mixed tocotrienol. • 400 to 800 IU
BIOFLAVANOID COMPLEX OF ANTIOXIDANTS	Bioflavanoids offer a necessary variety of potent antioxidants and are a great asset to your supplements. The amounts may vary but should include the majority of the following: • Rutin • Quercetin • Broccoli • Green Tea • Cruciferous • Bilberry • Grape-Seed Extract • Bromelain
ALPHA-LIPOLIC ACID	• 15 to 30 mg
CoQ10	• 20 to 30 mg
GLUTATHIONE	• 10 to 20 mg • Precusor: N-acetyl-L-cysteine 50 to 75 mg
B VITAMINS (COFACTORS)	• Folic Acid 800 to 1000 mcg • Vitamin B1 (Thiamin) 20 to 30 mg • Vitamin B2 (Riboflavin) 25 to 50 mg • Vitamin B3 (Niacin) 30 to 75 mg • Vitamin B5 (Pantothenic Acid) 80 to 200 mg • Vitamin B6 (Pyridoxine) 25 to 50 mg • Vitamin B12 (Cobalamin) 100 to 250 mcg • Biotin 300 to 1,000 mcg

OTHER IMPORTANT VITAMINS
- Vitamin D3 (Cholecalciferol)----450 IU to 800 IU
- Vitamin K   50 to 100 mcg

MINERAL COMPLEX
- Calcium 800 to 1,500 mg depending on your dietary intake of calcium
- Magnesium----500 to 800 mg
- Zinc----20 to 30 mg
- Selenium----200 cg is ideal
- Chromium----200 to 300 mcg
- Copper----1 to 3 mg
- Manganese----3 to 6 mg
- Vanadium----30 to 100 mcg
- Iodine----100 to 200 mcg
- Molybdenum----50 to 100 mcg
- Mixture of Trace Minerals

ADDITIONAL NUTRIENTS FOR BONE HEALTH
- Silicon----3 mg
- Boron----2 to 3 mg

OTHER IMPORTANT AND ESSENTIAL NUTRIENTS
Improved Homocysteine levels and improved brain function
- Choline----100 to 200 mg
- Trimethylglycine----200 to 500 mg
- Inositol----150mg to 250 mg

Supplementing Your Diet

ESSENTIAL FATS:
- Cold-Pressed Flaxseed oil
- Fish Oil Capsules

FIBER SUPPLEMENT
- Blend of soluble and insoluble fiber----10 to 30 mg depending on your dietary consumption of fiber (ideal is 35 to 50 grams of total fiber daily)

** *Several nutritional companies are putting together these essential nutrients into one or two different tablets, which need to be taken 2 to 3 times daily in order to achieve this level of supplementation. Look for a high-quality product that comes as close as possible to these recommendations. If the manufacturer follows pharmaceutical GMP and USP guidelines, you will be giving yourself the absolute best protection against oxidative stress.*

The essential fats and fiber provide added nutrients that are usually missing in the Western diet.

nutrients to the cell *in a complete and balanced fashion*. Then and only then will the cell have everything it needs to operate at its optimal capacity.

Protecting Your Health

Nutritional supplementation is really about health, not disease. Attacking the root cause of chronic degenerative disease is true preventive medicine. I realize that most of my readers enjoy good health and want to continue. Although I have shared many stories about patients who have developed a serious illness and were able to take back control of their health again, everyone would agree that it's much easier to maintain health than it is to try to regain it.

By applying these same principles, you who are in good health can decrease the risk of developing these chronic degenerative diseases. And those of you who are struggling with your health can empower your body to fight, if not reverse, chronic disease. When you combine a healthy diet, modest exercise program, and cellular nutrition, you always win healthwise. Isn't this your goal?

The fact is, an apple a day won't keep the doctor away. Today you need to supplement your apple and the rest of your well-balanced diet with high-quality nutritional supplements. Here I want to advise you of the basic nutrients you need to provide optimal cellular nutrition for your body.

When you provide all of these nutrients at optimal levels, your body receives all the health benefits nutritional supplementation provides. LDL cholesterol is more resistant to oxidation. Homocysteine levels decrease. Your eyes have greater antioxidant protection from the sunlight. The lungs have optimal protection. You enhance your immune and antioxidant defense system. You decrease the risk of developing heart disease, stroke, cancer, macular degeneration, cataracts, arthritis, Alzheimer's dementia, Parkinson's disease, asthma, diabetes, MS, lupus, and more.

Remember, this toxic world combined with our stressful lifestyle make it imperative that our immune system and antioxidant defense system are firing on all cylinders.

Optimizers

Sometimes a patient needs more than those nutrients listed in Table 1. If a patient is suffering from lasting fatigue or a chronic degenerative disease, he is under even more oxidative stress than normal, so I add what I call *optimizers* to his supplement program. These are antioxidants that are proven to be extremely potent. Nutritional companies are continually looking for more and more potent antioxidants, but presently the best is grape-seed extract, which is loaded with proanthacyanidins. These are very potent antioxidants that fall in a group of antioxidants called bioflavanoids, found in the colorful parts of fruits.

Grape-seed extract offers antioxidants that are fifty times more potent than vitamin E and twenty times more potent than vitamin C when used with all of the other antioxidants and supporting nutrients. Used alone, it is only six to seven times more potent than vitamin E and three to four times more potent than vitamin C. Here again the power of synergy among nutrients is clear.

Don't forget one of the most important characteristics of grape-seed extract—the fact that it crosses through the blood brain barrier easily (see Chapter 13). In other words it gets into the fluid around the brain, spinal cord, and nerves most readily. For fatigued patients I usually recommend adding at least 100–200 mg of grape-seed extract, depending on the severity of their problem. It usually will only take four to six weeks before my patients are able to notice a significant improvement and feel normal again. They can actually back off their optimizers at this point, as long as they continue to do well.

Patients who are already suffering from a chronic degenerative disease such as MS, heart disease, lupus, Crohn's, cancer, or Parkinson's, are already in serious trouble. In this setting even normal, everyday free-radical production causes significant oxidative damage to fats, proteins, and the DNA of the cell. The repair systems are so overwhelmed they simply are not able to keep up and repair all of this damage. These patients need significantly more potent antioxidants if they are to have any hope of "capturing" their disease and redeeming their health. Again, in this situation, I also recommend optimizers be added to the basic cellular nutritional program recommended in Table 1.

The first optimizer I will usually choose is grape-seed extract, but for those struggling with chronic disease I will usually recommend much higher doses than I would for patients with just fatigue. Other optimizers would be CoQ10, glucosamine sulfate, lutein, zeaxanthine, niacin, magnesium, and calcium.

Following are the basic principles and nutrients I use as optimizers in these various chronic degenerative diseases. All of my patients are taking the nutrients detailed in Table 1. I then add additional optimizers to this basic cellular nutrition program according to the seriousness of each individual case. Other than grape-seed extract, the optimizer I recommend most is CoQ10. It is not only a potent antioxidant but it is also essential for the creation of energy within the cell. In addition CoQ10 is a very important nutrient in enhancing the immune system.

[Note: CoQ10 is difficult to absorb. I am giving levels for the powder form in the following recommendations. You would need less CoQ10 if you take the Q-gel or soft-gel form of CoQ10]

Specific Optimizers I Recommend Be Added to the Nutrients in Table 1 for Each of These Particular Diseases

Heart Disease

I add approximately 100 mg each of grape-seed extract and CoQ10 along with some additional magnesium, about 200 to 300 mg per day. I feel it is critical for these patients to be taking a basic product that contains a mixture of vitamin Es as mentioned in Table 1.

If one's homocysteine level does not drop below 7 with just the B vitamins listed in Table 1, I will add 1–5 g of TMG (trimethylglycine) to the patient's regimen.

Cardiomyopathy

I add 300–600 mg of CoQ10 to a patient's regimen along with some additional magnesium and 100 mg grape-seed extract. Patients will usually see a response within 4 months. CoQ10 is very safe and the top researchers in the country feel comfortable pushing to 600 mg daily if the patient is not responding to the lower doses. However, some cardiologists like to perform blood level testing on the amount of CoQ10 in your blood before they begin to push to these higher levels.[1]

Cancer Patients

It is hard to give a simple formula for all the various cancers. But if there is no evidence of the cancer spreading (or the surgeon believes he totally removed it), I will add 200 mg each of grape-seed extract and CoQ10. If the patient has metastatic cancer (cancer that's spread), I will recommend 300 mg of grape-seed extract along with 500–600 mg of CoQ10. Children ages 8 to 15 should take only half of the recommended levels on Table 1 and half of the grape-seed extract and CoQ10 recommended here.

Macular Degeneration

For patients with this condition, I primarily add 300 mg of grape-seed extract to the nutrients found in Table 1. I also add approximately 6–12 mg of additional lutein to the regime. I have found that if these patients are going to improve, it will occur within the first 4 months.

Multiple Sclerosis

My patients with MS have shown that at least 400 mg of grape-seed extract, 200–300 mg of CoQ10, and even some additional 500 to 1000 mg of vitamin C can be helpful in this disease. I warn my MS patients that it may be more than 6 months before they see any improvement.

Lupus and Crohn's Disease

These patients need about 300 mg of grape-seed extract and 200 mg of CoQ10 added to the basic supplements. Again, if these patients improve, it's usually after about 6 months.

Osteoarthritis

I add 1,500–2,000 mg of glucosamine sulfate and about 100–200 mg of grape-seed extract. I have no problem if they also add 400 to 600 mg chondroitin sulfate or even 100 mg of MSM if the patients feel these help. I do not feel the medical evidence is strong enough at this time to absolutely recommend them as optimizers.

Rheumatoid Arthritis

Again I add 1,500–2000 mg of glucosamine sulfate, 300 mg of CoQ10, 400 mg of grape-seed extract, and 200 mg of additional magnesium and calcium. And I increase the omega-3 fatty acids by adding 3 to 4 fish oil capsule or two teaspoons of cold-pressed flax seed daily.

Osteoporosis

For these patients I do not recommend adding optimizers to my recommendations on Table 1; however, I strongly encourage them to be getting the right levels of vitamin D, calcium, and magnesium and to be sure they are taking these with food. They also need to get involved in an aggressive weight-bearing exercise program for the upper body.

Asthma

I add 200–300 mg of grape-seed extract (children should take about 2 mg per pound per day) along with additional 1,000 mg vitamin C (children: 200–500 milligrams), and 200 mg magnesium (children could add an additional 100 mg).

Emphysema

The basic nutrients in Table 1 are usually sufficient. I also may add 200 mg of grape-seed extract along with additional vitamin C and magnesium as indicated above under asthma.

Alzheimer's Dementia and Parkinson's Disease

As I mentioned earlier, these patients have already lost a significant number of brain cells before the diagnosis is even made. I have seen some significant improvement with Parkinson's disease, though if the patient starts an aggressive nutritional program early in his disease. I recommend adding 400 mg of grape-seed extract to the regimen on Table 1. There is good medical evidence that the progression of the Alzheimer's disease and Parkinson's disease may be slowed with this regimen.[2]

Diabetes Mellitus

I add approximately 100–200 mg of additional grape-seed extract to this regime. The cellular nutrition listed on Table 1 definitely provides everything else the body needs.

Chronic Fatigue/ Fibromyalgia

I add 200–300 mg of grape-seed extract along with 100–200 mg of CoQ10 to the basic supplement program. Sometimes I need to increase the grape-seed extract to 400 or even 500 mg daily in order to capture this disease. Once patients are responding favorably, the amount can be decreased to a lower maintenance level.

Need More Help?

These recommendations may seem overly simple to you. Yet these are the principles I have used to achieve the results I have shared with you in this book. It is not within the scope of this book to share with you my specific recommendations for each and every disease. I refer you to my web page at *www.nutritional-medicine.net* to get specific advice for the disease in which you are most interested.

On my web page I spell out recommendations in much greater detail; these are what I have used in my medical practice for more than fifty of these chronic degenerative diseases. I also offer, for a reasonable charge, individual e-mail nutritional consultations for those who wish to contact me directly. If you become a member of my web page, you'll have unlimited access to the web page, receive my bimonthly newsletter, and pay reduced consultation fees.

Choosing Your Nutritional Supplements

My purpose in writing this book is not to recommend any particular brand or type of nutritional supplements. But there are a few basic guidelines you need to follow in order to assure that you are taking high-quality supplements. I strongly recommend that you do not simply sell your health to the lowest bidder. Once you finally become convinced that nutritional supplements can offer you a health benefit, you want to be sure you are getting what you pay for.

You will not get the optimal results I share in this book when you take low-quality supplements. As you will learn, this is a poorly regulated industry. It will take some effort on your part to check out the quality of a particular product you choose to buy. But it is critical that you purchase high-quality supplements that are complete and balanced, if you are going to have any chance to protect or redeem your health.

As in any industry, the raw products used and how these products are manufactured affect their quality. I now advise my patients to purchase the best quality of supplement they can afford. Everyone needs to assess the importance of his or her health and what value he or she places on it. I realize that this can be a significant economic decision for most people. I look at nutritional supplements as my health insurance. Once you lose your health, it is very difficult to regain it, no matter how much money you are willing and able to spend.

When you look at my basic recommendations found on Table 1, you will quickly realize that you cannot get this amount of supplementation in a simple daily multivitamin. You need to choose a supplement that is as complete and balanced as possible. Several companies are now putting all of these nutrients together in one or two different pills. In order to achieve these optimal levels, however, you will most likely need to take several (four to eight tablets) daily. The more antioxidants and the more varied the antioxidants your supplement provides, the better. You must also be sure that you are getting all the minerals and B-cofactors.

You need to spend a little time investigating the nutritional company you choose. You can locate a lot of information on the company's website, or you may need to call the company directly. The most important thing to find out is whether the particular company you choose follows Good Manufacturing Practices (GMP) for pharmaceuticals. These companies produce what is called *pharmaceutical-grade supplements*. This means the company follows similar guidelines for producing its products as companies making over-the-counter drugs. The government does not require companies to do this, however some companies want to give their customers the assurance that they are getting what they are paying for by producing a high quality, pharmaceutical-grade product.

These high-quality manufacturers will put the actual amounts of the nutrients found in their products on the label and give full disclosure of all their ingredients. You may also find an expiration date on the bottle (this is really nice) and the company's full address. An encouraging sign is an actual street address rather than a P.O. box.

Another aspect to look for when you are researching a particular company is where it markets its products. A company marketing internationally usually has to follow higher standards than those companies who market only in the U.S. Canada, Australia, and Western European countries have the highest standards for the manufacturing of nutritional supplements. Some of these countries will also periodically send officials to perform on-site inspections of these manufacturing plants. It is really nice if the company is able to show you a third-party certification documenting the quality of its manufacturing practices.

Does all of this sound too picky? The November 1997 Tufts University Newsletter reported a study at the University of Maryland that looked carefully at nine different prescription prenatal vitamins. They did not look at what was in them but instead looked to see if they even dissolved. (If the pill doesn't even dissolve, it doesn't really matter what is in it.) They discovered that only three of the nine prenatal vitamins even dissolved. That is correct: only three of the nine. The pills that dissolved were produced under what are called U.S. Pharmacopoeia (USP) standards.

These are government guidelines that assure you and me that medications and supplement tablets will be absorbed by our bodies. Pharmaceutical GMPs are worthless if the company does not also follow USP standards for the dissolution of its tablets. Choosing a company that follows the USP guidelines is certainly a step in the right direction.

Sometimes it is quite difficult to find out information about the quality control that various companies use in their manufacturing process. The number of nutritional supplements that are available on the market today alone may overwhelm you. Every company is trying to find its niche in this very competitive market. Look through the marketing hype and try to get to the heart of the completeness and the quality of their nutritional products. Hopefully, these guidelines will help.

●　　●　　●

If you were to put all of the medical advances made since the beginning of recorded history into a twenty-four-hour time period, the medical evidence presented in this book would have occurred within the last five or six seconds. This is cutting-edge medical research. Most physicians and health-care practitioners have yet to come on board and make this research practical for the average, everyday person.

Be that as it may, the simple concept of cellular nutrition is the best way to defend yourself from the underlying threat of oxidative stress. By combining a healthy diet, a modest exercise program, and cellular nutrition, you are giving yourself the absolute best chance to protect your health or to redeem it after it has been lost. You have learned the power of complementary medicine.

The wide variety of true clinical stories presented in this book demonstrates the amazing healing power our bodies possess. The patients whose stories I have shared with you still have their underlying diseases, and many are still taking a significant amount of medication; yet they are living life to its fullest. When physicians take advantage of this most tremendous asset, the host—our bodies—and support it rather than deny its importance in the healing process, phenomenal clinical improvement is possible.

Tricia Rhodes, in her powerful book titled *Taking Up Your Cross*, shares a profound and fitting piece of wisdom for us here: "Always remember the brevity of life, the certainty of death, and the length of eternity."[3] We are not going to live forever in these "earth suits." They will wear out, and one day our full redemption will draw nigh. But in the meantime, these health concepts are the best way to care for and protect our health. And may we all *live* until we die.

Notes and Bibliography

Introduction

1. A. Zuger, "Fever Pitch: Getting Doctors to Prescribe Is Big Business," *New York Times*, 11 January 1999, A1, A3.

2. Ibid.

3. Matthew 9:12

4. M. R. Greenwood, "Doctors need more nutrition training," *American Journal of Clinical Nutrition*, (1998), 68.

Chapter 1

1. K. Cooper, *The Antioxidant Revolution* (Nashville: Thomas Nelson, 1994), 54–63.

2. Calvin Davies, "Oxidative stress: The paradox of aerobic life," *Biochem Soc Symp*, 61 (1995), 1-31.

3. Cooper.

Chapter 2

1. *Historical Statistics of the United States: Colonial Times to 1970*, U.S. Department of Commerce, Bureau of the Census, 58.

2. *Health in the United States: 1996-1997* (Department of Health and Human Services, 1997).

3. *Health Care Statistics* (Organization for Economic Cooperation and Development, 1992).

4. K.G. Kinsella, *American Journal of Clinical Nutrition*, 55 (1992).

5. *Health in the United States*.

6. Ibid.

7. P. Kovacic, "Mechanisms of carcinogenesis: Focus on oxidative stress," *Current Med Chemistry*, 8 (2001), 773-796.

8. Surgeon General's report on physical activity and health reported by the Center for Disease Control. Located at www..cdc.gov/nccdphp/sgr/chapcon.htm.

Chapter 3

1. ATP is the abbreviation for adenosine triphosphate.
2. Anthony Diplock, Antioxidant nutrients and disease prevention: an overview, *American Journal of Clinical Nutrition* 53, 1 (January 1991 [supplement]): 189S-93S
3. Cooper.
4. 20th U. S. Public Health Services Report released in 1986 by C. Everet Koop, M. D.
5. Ibid.
6. N. Seppa, "Secondary Smoke Carries High Price," *Science News Online*, 17 January 1998, *www.sciencenews.org/sn_arc98/1_17_98/fob* 1.htm.
7. Peter Moller, H. Wallin, and L. Knudsen, "Oxidative stress associated with exercise, psychological stress, and lifestyle factors," *Chemico-Biological Interactions*, 102 (1996), 17-36.
8. Ibid.
9. D. Bates, M.D., "Incidence of adverse drug events and potential adverse drug events," *JAMA*, 274 (1995), 29-34.

Additional References

McCord, Joe. "The evolution of free radical and oxidative stress." *American Journal of Medicine*, 108 (2000), 652-659.

Sacheck, J.M. "Role of vitamin E and oxidative stress in exercise." *Nutrition*, 17 (2001), 809-814.

Sohal, R.S. "Current issues concerning the role of oxidative stress in aging: A perspective."

Stohs, S.J. "The role of free radicals in toxicity and disease." *Journal of Basic and Clinical Physiology and Pharmacology*, 6 (1995), 205-228.

Chapter 4

1. K. Davies, "Oxidative stress, antioxidant defenses, and damage removal, repair, and replacement systems," *Life*, 50 (2000), 279-289.
2. Ibid.
3. Psalm 139:14
4. Davies, "Oxidative stress, antioxidant defenses."
5. Eric Schlosser, *Fast Food Nation* (Houghton Mifflin, 2001).

Additional References

Elsayed, N.M. "Antioxidant mobilization in response to oxidative stress: A dynamic environmental-nutritional interaction." *Nutrition*, 17 (2000), 828.

Young I.S. "Antioxidants in health and disease." *Journal of Clinical Pathology*, 54 (2001), 176-186.

Chapter 5

1. P.C. Ridker, "Reactive protein and other markers of inflammation in the prediction of cardiovascular disease in women," *New England Journal of Medicine*, 342.

2. National Cholesterol Education Program, *Second Report of the Expert Panel on Detection, Evaluation, and Treatment of High Blood Cholesterol in Adults* (Bethesda, MD: National Heart, Lung, and Blood Institute, 1993).

3. Daniel Steinberg, M.D.; Sampath Parthasarathy, Ph.D.; Thomas Carew, Ph.D., et al., "Beyond cholesterol: Modifications of low-density lipoprotein that increase its atherogenicity," *New England Journal of Medicine*, 320 (1989), 915-924.

4. *Health in the United States.*

5. R. Ross, "Atherosclerosis: An inflammatory disease," *New England Journal of Medicine*, 340 (1999), 115-123.

6. Daniel Steinberg, M.D., Ph.D., "Antioxidants in the prevention of human atherosclerosis," Summary of the proceedings of a National Heart, Lung, and Blood Institute workshop: September 5-6, 1991.

7. B. Frei, "On the role of vitamin C and other antioxidants in the atherogenesis and vascular dysfuntion," *Proc Soc Exp Biol Med*, 222 (1999), 196-204.

8. J.M. May, "How does ascorbic acid prevent endothelial dysfunction?" *Free Radic Biol Med*, 28 (2000), 1421-1429.

   And

   N. Gokce, "Long term ascorbic acid administration reserves endothelial vasomotor dysfunction in patients with coronary artery disease,"99 (1999), 3234-3240.

9. S. Lenhart, "Vitamins for management of cardiovascular disease," *Pharmaco*, 19 (1999), 1400-1414.

10. B. Fuhrman, "Flavanoids protect LDL from oxidation and attenuate atherosclerosis," *Current Opin Lipidol*, 12 (2001), 41-48.

11. J. Stein, "Purple grape juice improves endothelial function and reduces susceptibility of LDL cholesterol to oxidation in patients with coronary artery disease," *Circulation*, 100 (1999), 1050-1055.

Additional References

Carr, A. "The role of natural antioxidants in preserving the biological activity of endothelium-derived nitric oxide." *Free Radic Biol Med.*, 28 (2000), 1806-1814.

Davies, K. "Oxidative stress, antioxidant defenses, and damage removal, repair, and replacement systems." *Life*, 50 (2000), 279-289.

Diaz, M.N., et al. "Antioxidants and atherosclerotic heart disease." *New England Journal of Medicine*, 337 (1997), 408-416.

Forgione, M.A. "Roles of endothelial dysfunction in coronary artery disease." *Current Opinions in Cardiology*, 15 (2000), 409-415.

Harris, W. "The prevention of atherosclerosis with antioxidants." *Cardiology*, 640 (1992).

Hennekens, C.H. "Antioxidants and heart disease: Epidemiology and clinical evidence." *Clinical Cardiology*, 16 (1993), 10-15.

Hodis, M.D., Howard N., et al. "Serial coronary angiographic evidence that antioxidant vitamin intake reduces progression of coronary artery atherosclerosis." *JAMA*, 273 (1995), 1849-1854.

Koenig, W. "Inflammation and coronary heart disease: An overview." *Cardiology Review*, 9 (2001), 31-35.

Merchant, N. "Oxidative stress in cardiovascular disease." *Journal of Nucl Cardiology*, 8 (2001), 379-389.

Morris, PhD., M.D., D.L., et al. "Serum carotenoids and coronary artery disease." *JAMA*, 272 (1994), 1439-1441.

Ross, Ph.D., R., and J.A. Glomset, M.D. "The pathogenesis of atherosclerosis." *New England Journal of Medicine*, 295 (1996), 369-375.

Stampfer, M.D., Meir J.; Charles H. Hennekens, M.D., et al. "Vitamin E consumption and the risk of coronary disease in women." *New England Journal of Medicine*, 328 (1993), 1444-1449.

Tardiff, J.C. "Insights into oxidative stress and atherosclerosis." *Can J Cardiol*, 16 (2000), 2D-4D.

Chapter 6

1. C.J. Boushey, S.A. Beresford, G.S. Omen, A.G. Motulsky, "A quantitative assessment of plasma homocysteine as a risk factor for vascular disease," *JAMA*, 274 (1995), 1049-1057.

2. K. McCully, *The Homocysteine Revolution* (Keats Publishing, 1997).

3. M. Stacey, "The Rise and Fall of Kilmer McCully," *New York Times*, August 1997.

4. Ibid.

5. Ibid.

6. M.J. Stampfer, M.R. Manilow, W.C. Willett, et al., "A prospective study of plasma homocyst(e)ine and risk of myocardial infarction in US physicians," *JAMA*, 268 (1992), 877-881.

7. Jacob Selhub, Ph.D.; P.F. Jacques, et al., "Association between plasma homocysteing concentrations and extracranial carotid artery stenosis," *New England Journal of Medicine*, 332 (1995), 286-291.

8. I.M. Graham, L.E. Daly, et al., "Plasma homocysteine as a risk factor for vascular disease," *JAMA*, 277 (1997), 1775-1781.

9. Stacey.

10. Ibid.

11. Ibid.

12. Ibid.

13. Ibid.

14. Stacey.

15. Ibid.

Additional References

Calvaca, V. "Oxidative stress and homocysteine in coronary artery disease." *Clinical Chemistry*, 47 (2001), 887-892.

Eickelboom, J. "Homocysteine and cardiovascular disease." *Annals of Internal Medicine*, 131 (1999), 363-375.

Maxwell, S.R. "Coronary artery disease-free radical damage, antioxidant protection and the role of homocysteine." *Basic Res Cardiol*, 95 (2000), 165-171.

McBride, P. "Hyperhomocyst(e)inemia and atherosclerotic vascular disease." *Arch Intern Med*, 158 (1998), 1301-1306.

Moghadadsian, M. "Homocysteine and coronary artery disease." *Arch Internal Medicine*, 157 (1997).

Ridker, P.C. "Reactive protein and other markers of inflammation in the prediction of cardiovascular disease in women." *New England Journal of Medicine*, 342.

Tice, J. "Cost effectiveness of vitamin therapy to lower plasma homocysteine levels for the prevention of coronary heart disease." *JAMA*, 286 (2001).

Yeun, J.Y. "C reactive protein, oxidative stress, homocysteine, and troponin as inflammatory and metabolic predictors of atherosclerosis in ESRD." *Current Opinion Nephrol Hypertension*, 9 (2000), 621-630.

Chapter 7

1. H. Langsjoen, P. Langsjoen, et al., "Usefulness of coenzyme Q10 in clinical cardiology: A long-term study," *Molecular Aspects of Medicine*, 15 (1994), 165-175.

2. P.H. Langsjoen, A.M. Langsjoen, "Overview of the use of CoQ10 in cardiovascular disease," *Biofactors*, 9 (1999), 273-284.

3. Ibid.

4. K. Folkers, P. Langsjoen, P.H. Langsjoen, "Therapy with coenzyme Q10 of patients in heart failure who are eligible or ineligible for a transplant," *Biochem Biophys Res Commun*, 182 (1992), 247-253.

5. E. Baggio, R. Gandini, et al., "Italian multi-center study on the safety and efficacy of coenzyme Q10 as adjunctive therapy in heart failure," *Molecular Aspects of Medicine*, 15 (1994), 287-294.

6. Folkers.

7. Ibid.

8. Stephen Sinatra, M.D., *The Coenzyme Q10 Phenomenon* (Keats, 1998), 37.

9. P.H. Langsjoen, K. Folkers, "A six-year clinical study of therapy of cardiomyopathy with coenzyme Q10," *International Journal of Tissue Reactions*, 12 (1990), 169-171.

10. Langsjoen, "Usefulness."

11. Sinatra.

12. A special-use patent can be obtained; however, as long as the product can be purchased over the counter, it has no value.

13. Langsjoen, "A six-year study."

Additional References

Folkers, K. "Lovastatin decreases conenzyme Q levels in humans." *Proc National Acadademy Sci USA*, 87 (1990), 8931-8934.

Langsjoen, P.H.; K. Folkers, et al. "Effective and safe therapy with coenzyme Q10 for cardiomyopathy." *Klinische Wochenschrift*, 66 (1988), 583-590.

Witte, K.K. "Chronic heart failure and micronutrients." *Journal of the American College of Cardiology*, 37 (2001), 1765-1774.

Chapter 8

1. *Health in the United States.*
2. P. Kovacic, "Mechanisms of carcinogenesis: Focus on oxidative stress," *Current Med. Chemistry*, 8 (2001), 773-796.
3. Ibid.
4. Ibid.
5. Tom Paulson, "Seattle Biochemist Challenging Cancer Theories," *Seattle Post-Intelligencer*, 26 November 1996.
6. Kovacic.
7. Paulson.
8. Ibid.
9. Kovacic.
10. Ibid.
11. G. Block, "Dietary guidelines and the results of food surveys," *American Journal of Clinical Nutrition*, 53 (1991), 3565-3575.
12. Ibid.
13. R. Voelker, "Ames agrees with Mom's advice: Eat your fruits and vegetables," *JAMA*, 273 (1995), 1077-1078.
14. Ibid.
15. S.J. Duthie, M.A. Aiguo, M.A. Ross, and A.R. Collins, "Antioxidant supplementation decreases oxidative DNA damage in human lymphocytes," *Cancer Research*, 15 (1996), 1291-1295.

    And

    Hartmann, A.M. Niess, et al., "Vitamin E prevents exercise-induced DNA damage," *Mutation Research*, 348 (1995), 195-202.
16. H.S. Garewal, "Chemoprevention of cancer," *Hematol Oncol Clin North Am*, 1 (1991), 69-77.
17. G. Shklar, J. Schwartz, et al., "The effectiveness of a mixture of beta-carotene, alphatochopherol, glutathione, and ascorbic acid for cancer prevention," *Nutrition and Cancer*, 20 (1993), 145-151.
18. V. Singh, "Premalignant lesions' role of antioxidant vitamins and B carotene is risk reduction and prevention of malignant transformation," *American Journal of Clinical Nutrition*, 53 (1991), 386-390.

    And

S.L. Romney, et al., "Nutrient antioxidants in the pathogenesis and prevention of cervical dysplasia and cancer," *J Scell Biochem Suppl*, 23 (1995), 96-103.

19. Romney.

20. K. Prasad, "High doses of multiple antioxidant vitamins," *Journal of the American College of Nutrition*, 18 (1999), 13-25.

21. Ibid.

22. K. Lockwood, S. Moesgaard, and K. Folkers, "Partial and complete regression of breast cancer in patients in relation to dosage of coenzyme Q10," *Biochemical and Biophysical Research Communications*, 199 (1994), 1504-1508.

Additional References

Conklin, K. "Dietary antioxidants during cancer chemotherapy." *Nutrition and Cancer*, 37 (2000), 1-18.

Davies, K. "Oxidative stress, antioxidant defenses, and damage removal, repair, and replacement systems." *Life*, 50 (2000), 279-289.

Hahn, S. "New directions for free radical cancer research and medical applications." *Free Radicals in Diagnostic Medicine*, 1994.

Chapter 9

1. ARMD Study Group, "Multicenter ophthalmic and nutritional ARMD study, part one: Design, subjects, and procedures," *Journal of the American Optometry Association*, 67 (1996), 12-29.

2. A. Taylor, "Effect of photooxidation on the eye lens and role of nutrients in delaying cataract," *EXS*, 62 (1992), 266-279.

3. S.D. Varma, "Prevention of cataracts by nutritional and metabolic antioxidants," *Crit Rev Food Sci Nutr*, 35 (1995), 111-129.

4. H. Taylor, "2001 assessment of nutritional influences on risk for cataract," *Nutrition*, 10 (2001), 845-857.

5. P. Knekt, et al., "Serum antioxidant vitamins and risk of cataract," *British Medical Journal*, 305 (1992), 1392-1394.

6. P.F. Jacques, "The potential preventive effects of vitamins for cataract and age-related macular degeneration," *Int J Vitam Nutr Res*, 69 (1999), 198-205.

7. H. Heseker, "Antioxidant vitamins and cataracts in the elderly," *Zeitschrift Fur Ernahrungswissenschaft*, 34 (1995), 167-176.

8. F. Giblin, "Glutathione: A vital lens antioxidant," *J Ocular Pharm*, 16 (2000).

9. L.M. Jampol, F.L. Ferris, "Antioxidants and zinc to prevent progression of age-related macular degeneration," *JAMA*, 286 (2001), 2466-2468.

10. Van Der Hagen, "Free radicals and antioxidant supplementation: A review of their roles in age related macular degeneration," *J Am Optom Assoc*, 64 (1993), 871-878.

11. Ibid.

12. Eye Disease Case-Control Study Group, "Antioxidant status and neovascular age-related macular degeneration," *Arch Ophthalmol*, 111 (1993), 1499.

13. J.T. Landrum, et al., "A one year study of the macular pigment: The effect of 140 days of a lutein supplement," *Exp Eye Res*, 65 (1997), 57-62.

14. P.S. Bernstein, "Identification and quantification of carotenoids and their metabolites in the tissue of the human eye," *Exp Eye Res*, 722 (2001), 15-23.

15. B.S. Winkler, M.E. Boulton, et al., "Oxidative damage and age-related macular degeneration," *Molecular Vision*, 5 (1999), 32.

16. Ibid.

17. M.A. Blasi, C. Bovina, et al., "Does coenzyme Q10 play a role in opposing oxidative stress inpatients with age-related macular degeneration?" *Ophthalmologica*, 215 (2001), 51-54.

18. Winkler.

19. Ibid.

20. Jampol.

21. Van Der Hagen.

Additional References

Delcourt, C. "Age related macular degeneration and antioxidant status in the POLA study." *Arch Opthalmol.*, 117 (1999), 1384-1390.

Marak, G.E., et al. "Free radicals and antioxidants in the pathogenesis of eye diseases." *Advances in Experimental Medicine and Biology*, 264 (1990), 513-527.

Robertson, J.M., et al. "Vitamin E intake and risk of cataracts in humans." *Annals of the New York Academy of Science*, 570 (1989), 372-382.

Varma, S. "Scientific basis for medical therapy of cataracts by antioxidants." *American Journal of Clinical Nutrition*, 53 (1991), 335-345.

Chapter 10

1. K. Schmidt, "Interaction of antioxidative micronutrients with host defense mechanisms: A critical review," *Internat J Vit Nutr Res*, 67 (1997), 307-311.

2. R.P. Tengerdy, et al., "Vitamin E immunity and disease resistance," *Diet and Resistance to Disease* (New York: Plenum Press, 1981).

    And

    Schmidt.

3. K.R. Chandra, "Effect of vitamin and trace element supplementation on immune responses and infection in elderly subjects," *Lancet*, 340 (1992), 1124-1127.

4. Schmidt.

5. Ibid.

6. E. Bliznakov, "Coenzyme Q, the immune system, and aging," *New England Institute*.

    And

    E. Bliznakov, "Coenzyme Q in experimental infections and neoplasia," *New England Institute*, 1997.

7. G.A. Ebeby, et al., "Reduction in duration of common colds by zinc gluconate lozenges in a double-blind study," *Antimicorbial Agents and Chemotherapy*, 25 (1984), 20-24.

8. Chandra.

9. Ibid.

10. I.K. Mohan, "Oxidant stress, antioxidants, and essential fatty acids in systemic lupus erythemetosis," *No journal*, 56 (1997), 193-198.

11. A. Davidson, "Autoimmune diseases," *New England Journal of Medicine*, 345 (2001).

12. R. Vestn, "Active forms of oxygen and pathogenesis of rheumatoid arthritis and systemic lupus erythemetosis," *Vestn Ross Akad Nauk*, 12 (1996), 15-20.

   And

   G. Simonini, "Emerging potentials for an antioxidant therapy as a new approach to the treatment of systemic sclerosis," *Toxicology*, 155 (2000), 1-15.

   And

   G.W. Comstock, et al., "Serum concentrations of alpha-tocopherol, beta-carotene, and retinal preceding the diagnosis of rheumatoid arthritis and systemic lupus erythemetosis," *Annals of Rheumatic Diseases*, 56 (1997), 323-325.

13. Ibid.

Additional References

Babior, B. "Phagocytes and oxidative stress." *Excerpta Medica*, (2000).

Beharka, A. "Vitamin status and immune function." *Methods Enzymol*, 282 (1997), 247-263.

Biesalski, H.K. "Antioxidants in nutrition and their importance in the anti-/oxidative balance in the immune system." *Immun Infekt*, 23 (1995), 166-173.

Grimble, R.F. "Effect of antioxidative vitamins on immune function with clinical applications." *International Journal of Vitamin and Nutrition Res*, 67 (1997), 312-320.

Horowitz, J. "The Battle Within." *Time*, January 2002, 69-75.

Koch, T. "Total antioxidant capacity of colon in patients with chronic ulcerative colitis." *Digestive Diseases and Science*, 45 (2000).

Kubena, K.S. "Nutrition and the immune system." *Journal of the American Dietary Association*, 96 (1996), 1156-1164.

Kubes, P. "Nitric oxide and intestinal inflammation." *American Journal of Medicine*, 109 (2000), 150-158.

Wendland, B.E. "Lipid peroxidation and plasma antioxidant micronutrients in Crohn's disease." *American Journal of Clinical Nutrition*, 74 (2001), 259-264.

Chapter 11

1. *Harrison's Principles of Medicine, 14th edition* (McGraw and Hill 1935).

2. R. Miesel, et al., "Enhanced mitochondria! radical production in patients with rheumatoid arthritis correlates with elevated levels of tumor necrosis factor alpha in plasma," *Free Radical Research*, 25 (1996), 161-169.

3. M. Heliovaara, P. Knekt, et al., "Serum antioxidants and risk of rheumatoid arthritis," *Ann Rheum Dis*, 53 (1994), 51-53.

4. Ibid.

5. A. Drovanti, "Therapeutic activity of oral glucosamine sulfate in osteoarthritis," *Clin Ther*, 3 (1980), 260-272.

6. J.Y. Reginster, "Glucosamine sulfate significantly reduces progression of knee osteoarthritis over three years," The American College of Rheumatology, 63rd annual meeting.

7. T.E. McAlindon, M.P. LaValley, "Glucosamine and chondroitin for treatment of osteoarthritis," *JAMA*, 283 (2000), 1469-1475.

   And

   G. Qiu, "Efficacy and safety of glucosamine sulfate versus ibuprofen in patients with knee osteoarthritis," 48 (1998), 469-474.

8. McAlindon.

9. A. Gaby, "Nutrients and osteoporosis," *Journal of Nutritional Medicine*, 1 (1990), 63-72.

   And

   B. Dawson, "Rates of bone loss in postmenopausal women randomly assigned to one of two dosages of vitamin D," *American Journal of Clinical Nutrition*, 61 (1995), 1140-1145.

10. Y. Zhang, et al., "Bone mass and the risk of breast cancer among menopausal women," *New England Journal of Medicine*, 336 (1997), 611-617.

11. For a thorough discussion about these and other problems women face during menopause, I would recommend that you read Dr. Christiane Northrup's book entitled *The Wisdom of Menopause*.

12. B. Dawson-Hughes, M.D., et al., "Effect of calcium and vitamin D supplementation on bone density in men and women sixty-five years of age or older," *New England Journal of Medicine*, 337 (1997), 670-676.

13. S. Abram, "Calcium metabolism in girls: Current dietary intakes lead to low rates of calcium absorption and retention during puberty," *American Journal of Clinical Nutrition*, 60 (1994), 729-743.

14. G.E. Abraham, "The importance of magnesium in the management of primary post-menopausal osteoporosis," *Journal of Nutritional Medicine*, 2 (1991), 165-178.

   And

   M.S. Seelig, "Magnesium deficiency with phosphate and vitamin D excess: Roland pediatric cardiovascular nutrition," *Cardiovascular Medicine*, 3 (1978), 637-677.

15. M.K. Thomas, et al., "Hypovitaminosis D in medical patients," *New England Journal of Medicine*, (1998).

16. A. Tomita, "Post-menopausal osteoporosis calcium study with vitamin K," *Clinical Endocrinology*, 19 (1971), 731-736.

17. R.N. Leach, A.M. Muenster, "Studies on the role of manganese on bone formation," *Journal of Nutrition*, 78 (1962), 51-56.

18. A.J. Greico, "Homocystinuria: Pathogenetic mechanisms," *American Journal of Medical Science*, 273 (1977), 120-132.

19. S. Meacham, "Effect of boron supplementation on blood and urinary calcium, magnesium, and phosphorus, and urinary boron in athletic and sedentary women."

20. O.S. Atik, "Zinc and senile osteoporosis," *Journal of the American Geriatric Society*, 31 (1983), 790-791.

Additional References

Comstock, G.W., et al. "Serum concentrations of alpha-tocopherol, beta-carotene, and retinal preceding the diagnosis of rheumatoid arthritis and systemic lupus erythematosus." *Annals of Rheumatic Diseases*, 56 (1997), 323-325.

Dijkmans, B.A. "Folate supplementation and methotrexate." *Br Journal of Rheumatology*, 34 (1995), 1172-1174.

Greenwald, R.A. "Oxygen radicals, inflammation and arthritis: Pathophysiological considerations and implications for treatment." *Semin Arthritis Rheum*, 20 (1991), 219-240.

Henrotin, Y., et al. "Active oxygen species, articular inflammation and cartilage damage." *Free Radicals and Aging*, 62 (1992), 308-322.

Johnston, Jr., M.D., C.C., et al. "Calcium supplementation and increases in bone mineral density in children." *New England Journal of Medicine*, 327 (1992), 82-87.

Packard, P.T. "Medical nutrition therapy for patients with osteoporosis." *Journal of the American Dietary Association*, 97 (1997), 414-417.

Rodriguez, C. "Estrogen replacement therapy and ovarian cancer mortality in a large prospective study of U.S. women." *JAMA*, 285 (2001), 1460-1465.

Chapter 12

1. P. Barnes, "Reactive oxygen species and airway inflammation," *Free Rad Biol and Med*, 9 (1990), 235-243.

2. A. Van der Vliet, "Oxidants, nitrosants, and the lung," *The American Journal of Medicine*, 109 (2000), 398-421.

3. Ibid.

4. W. MacNee, "Oxidants/antioxidants and chronic obstructive pulmonary disease: Pathogenesis to therapy," *Novartis Found Symp*, 234 (2001), 169-188.

5. B. Portal, "Altered antioxidant status and increased lipid peroxidation in children with cystic fibrosis," *American Journal of Clinical Nutrition*, 61 (1995), 843-847.

6. L.G. Wood, D.A. Fitzgerald, et al., "Oxidative stress in cystic fibrosis: Dietary and metabolic factors," *Journal of the American College of Nutrition*, 20 (2001), 157-165.

7. V. Hudson, "Rethinking cystic fibrosis pathology: The critical role of abnormal reduced glutathione transport caused by CFTR mutation," *Free Radical Biology and Medicine*, 30, 1440-1461.

Additional References

Barnes, P.J. "Potential novel therapies for chronic obstructive pulmonary disease." *Novartis Foundation Symposium*, 234 (2001), 255-267.

MacNee, W. "Oxidants/antioxidants and chronic obstructive pulmonary disease: Pathogenesis to therapy." *Novartis Foundation Symposium*, 234 (2001), 169-188.

Morcillo, E.J. "Oxidative stress and pulmonary inflammation." *Pharmacological Research*, 40 (1999), 393-404.

Chapter 13

1. "Parkinson Report," *National Parkinson Foundation, Inc.*, 18 (1997).

2. J. Knight, "Reactive oxygen species and the neurodegenerative diseases," *Ann Clin and Lab Sci*, 27 (1997).

3. Ibid.

4. L. Honig, "Apoptosis and neurologic disease," *The American Journal of Medicine*, 108 (2000), 317-330.

5. D.B. Carr, "Current concepts in the pathogenesis of Alzheimer's Disease," *The American Journal of Medicine*, 103 (1997), 3-9.

6. M.A. Smith, "Radical aging in Alzheimer's Disease," *Trends in Neuroscience*, 18 (1995), 341-342.

7. M.A. Sano, "Controlled trial of selegiline, alpha tocopheral, or both as treatment for Alzheimer's Disease," *New England Journal of Medicine*, 336 (1997), 1216-1221.

8. G. Yossi, "Oxidative stress induced neurodegenerative diseases: The need for antioxidants that penetrate the blood barrier," *Neuropharm*, 40 (2001), 959-975.

9. Ibid.

10. S.M. LeVine, "The role of reactive oxygen species in the pathogenesis of multiple sclerosis," *Med Hypotheses*, 39 (1992), 271-274.

11. Ibid.

12. V. Calabrese, "Changes in cerebrospinal fluid levels of maliondialdehyde and glutathione reductase activity in multiple sclerosis," *Int J Clin PharmacolRes*, 14 (1994), 119-123.

13. Yossi.

14. Ibid.

15. Calabrese.

16. Yossi.

17. Ibid.

18. Ibid.

19. Ibid.

20. 2 Corinthians 5:8

Additional References

Beal, F. "Mitochondria, free radicals, and neurodegeneration." *Biology Ltd*, (1996).

Bo, L. "Induction of nitric oxide synthase in demyelinating regions of multiple sclerosis." *Annals of Neurology*, 36 (1994), 778-786.

Ceballos, P. "Peripheral antioxidant enzyme activities and selenium in elderly subjects and in dementia of Alzheimer type." *Free Radic Biol Med*, 20 (1996), 579-587.

Ebadi, M. "Oxidative stress and antioxidative therapy in Parkinson's disease." *Prog Neurobiol*, 48 (1996), 1-19.

Fahn, S. "An open trail of high-dosage antioxidants in early Parkinson's disease." *American Journal of Clinical Nutrition*, 53 (1991), 380-382.

Newcombe, J. "Low density lipoprotein uptake by macrophages in MS plaques: Implications for pathogenesis." *Neuropathol Appl Neurobiol*, 20 (1994), 152-162.

Prasad, K.N. "Multiple antioxidants in the prevention and treatment of neurodegenerative diseases." *Current Opinions in Neurology*, 12 (1999), 760-761.

Toshniwal, P.K. "Evidence for increased lipid peroxidation in MS." *Neurochem Research*, 17 (1992), 205-207.

Chapter 14

1. A.H. Mokdad, B.A. Bowman, et al., "The continuing epidemics of obesity and diabetes in the United States," *JAMA*, 286 (2001), 1195-1200.

2. R. Klein, et al., "Visual impairment and diabetes," *Ophthalmology*, 91 (1984), 1-9.

   And

   National Institute of Diabetes and Digestive and Kidney Diseases, "U.S. Renal Data System: 1994 Annual Data Report," Bethesda, 1994.

3. National Institute.

4. G. Reavens, *Syndrome X* (Simon and Schuster, 2000).

5. Ibid.

6. J.R. Margolis, et al., "Clinical features of unrecognized myocardial infarction: Silent and symptomatic. Eighteen-year follow up: The Framingham study," *American Journal of Cardiology*, 32 (1973), 1-7.

7. J. O'Keefe, "Improving adverse cardiovascular prognosis of type 2 diabetes," *Mayo Clin Proc*, 74 (1999), 171-180.

8. J. Brand-Miller, T.M. Wolever, et al., *The Glucose Revolution* (New York: Marlowe and Company, 1999), 26-27.

9. Ibid.

10. Walter Willet, *Eat, Drink, and Be Healthy* (Simon and Schuster, 2001).

11. P.A. Low, "The roles of oxidative stress and antioxidant treatment in experimental diabetic neuropathy," *Diabetes*, 46 (1997), 38-42.

12. Low.

    And

    R.A. Disilvestro, "Zinc in relation to diabetes and oxidative stress," *Journal of Nutritional Medicine*, 130 (2000), 1509-1511.

13. V.K. Liu, "Chromium and insulin in young subjects with normal glucose tolerance," *American Journal of Clinical Nutrition*, 35 (1982), 661-667.

14. G. Paolisso, "Daily magnesium supplements improve glucose handling in elderly subjects," *American Journal of Clinical Nutrition*, 55 (1992), 1161-1167.

Additional References

Defronzo, R. "Insulin resistance, hyperinsulinemia and coronary artery disease: A complex metabolic web." *Journal of Cardio Pharm*, 20 (1992), 1-16.

Gurler, B. "The role of oxidative stress in diabetic retinopathy." *Eye*, 14 (2000), 730-735.

Jakus, V. "The role of free radicals, oxidative stress and antioxidant systems in diabetic vascular disease." *Bratisl Lek Listy*, 101 (2000), 541-551.

McNair, M.D., P., et al. "Hypomagnesemia, a risk factor in diabetic retinopathy." *Diabetes*, 27 (1978), 1075-1077.

Sharma, A. "Effects of nonpharmacological intervention on insulin insensitivity." *Journal of Cardio Pharm*, 20 (1992), 27-34.

Wagner, E. "Effect of improved glycemic control on health care costs and utilization." *JAMA*, 285 (2001), 182-189.

Chapter 15

References

Bennett, R. "Myofascial pain and the chronic fatigue syndrome."

Eisinger, J. "Protein peroxidation magnesium deficiency and fibromyalgia." *Magnus Res*, 9 (1996), 313-316.

Keenoy, M. "Antioxidant status and lipoprotein peroxidation in chronic fatigue syndrome." *Life Csi*, 68 (2001), 2037-2049.

Logan, A.C. "Chronic fatigue syndrome: Oxidative stress and dietary modifications." *Alternative Medical Review*, 6 (2001), 450-459.

Chapter 16

1. R. Olson, ed., *Nutrition Reviews: Present Knowledge of Nutrition*, 6th ed. (Washington, DC: Nutrition Foundation, 1989), 96-107.

   And

   K.A. Munoz, et al., "Food intake of United States children and adolescents compared with recommendations," *Pediatrics*, 100 (1997), 323-329.

2. G. Block, "Dietary guidelines and the results of food surveys," *American Journal of Clinical Nutrition*, 53 (1991), 3565-3575.

3. F.E. Beach, et al., "Variation in mineral composition of vegetables," *Soil Science Society Proceedings*, 13 (1948), 380.

4. Ibid.

5. J. Lazarou, B.H. Pomeranz, P.N. Corey, "Incidence of adverse drug reactions in hospitalized patients," *JAMA*, 279 (1998).

6. M. Colgan, *The New Nutrition* (Apple Publishing, 1995) 10-15.

7. Lazarou.

8. Ibid.

9. K.J. Rothman, et al., "Teratogenecity of high vitamin A intake," *New England Journal of Medicine*, 333 (1995), 1369-1373.

10. M. Steiner, "Vitamin E: More than an antioxidant," *Clinical Cardiology*, 16 (1993), 16-18.

11. Murrah.

12. M.S. Seelig, "Magnesium deficiency with phosphate and vitamin D excess: Roland pediatric cardiovascular nutrition," *Cardiovascular Medicine*, 3 (1978), 637-650.

13. M.K. Thomas, "Hypovitaminosis D in medical patients," *New England Journal of Medicine*, (1998).

14. Ibid.

15. J.M. McKenney, et al., "A comparison of the efficacy and toxic effects of sustained-versus immediate-release niacin in hypercholesterolemic patients," *JAMA*, 271 (1994), 672-677.

16. G.J. Parry, D.E. Bredesen, "Sensory neuropathy with low-dose pyridoxine," *Neurology*, 35 (1985), 1466-1468.

17. Murrah.

18. NEJM article on calcium intake and kidney stones

19. Murrah.

20. Ibid.

21. Ibid.

22. Ibid.

23. A.N. Fan, K.W. Kizer, "Selenium: nutritional, toxicological and clinical aspects," *Western Journal of Medicine*, 153 (1990), 160-167.

24. Ibid.

25. Murrah.

26. Ibid.

27. D. Albanes, O.P. Heinonen, et al., "Alphatocopherol and beta-carotene supplements and lung cancer," *Journal of the National Cancer Institute*, 88 (1996).

28. O.S. Omen, G.E. Goodman, et al., "Effects of a combination of beta-carotene and vitamin A on lung cancer and cardiovascular disease," *New England Journal of Medicine*, 334 (1996), 1150-1155.

29. C.H. Hennekens, J.E. Buring, et al., "Lack of effect of long-term supplementation with beta-carotene on the incidence of malignant neoplasms and cariovasuclar disease," *New England Journal of Medicine*, 334 (1996), 1145-1149.

30. Albanes.

31. G.B. Brown, et al., "Simvastatin and niacin, antioxidant vitamins, or the combination for the prevention of coronary disease," *New England Journal of Medicine*, 345 (2001), 1583-1592.

Chapter 17

1. S.T. Sinatra, *The Coenzyme Q10 Phenomenon* (Keats Publishing, 1998), 33-47.

2. M.A. Sano, "Controlled trial of selegiline, alphatocopheral, or both as treatment for Alzheimer's Disease," *New England Journal of Medicine*, 336 (1997), 1216-1221.

    And

    L. Honig, "Apoptosis and neurologic disease," *The American Journal of Medicine*, 108 (2000), 317-330.

3. Tricia McCary-Rhodes, *Taking Up Your Cross* (Bethany Press International, 1998).

Additional References

Bagchi D. "Free radicals and grape seed proanthocyanidin extract: Importance in human health and disease prevention." *Toxicology*, 148 (2000),187-197.

Gaytan R. "Oral nutritional supplements and heart disease: A review." *Maer Journal of Therapy*, 8 (2001), 225-274.

Kontush A. "Lipophilic antioxidants in blood plasma as markers of atherosclerosis: The role of alpha-carotene and gamma-tocopherol." *Atherosclerosis*, 144 (1999), 117-122.

Obyrne D. "Studies of LDL oxidation following alpha, gamma, or delta tocotrienyl acetate supplementation of hypercholesterolemic humans." *Free Radical Biology and Medicine*, (2000).

Index

About the Author

RAY D. STRAND, M.D., GRADUATED FROM THE UNIVERSITY OF Colorado Medical School and finished his postgraduate training at Mercy Hospital in San Diego, California. He has been involved in an active private family practice for the past thirty years. He has focused his practice on nutritional medicine over the past seven years while lecturing internationally on the subject across the United States, Canada, Australia, England, and the Netherlands. Dr. Strand lives on a horse ranch in South Dakota with his lovely wife, Elizabeth. They have three grown children.

For more information on Dr. Strand's consulting and speaking services, you can contact Dr. Strand at:

Ray D. Strand, M. D.
P. O. Box 9226
Rapid City, SD 57709

Visit Dr. Strand's website:

www.nutritional-medicine.net

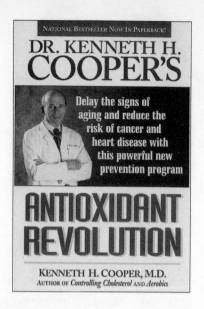

NATIONAL BESTSELLER NOW IN PAPERBACK!

DR. KENNETH H. COOPER'S

Delay the signs of aging and reduce the risk of cancer and heart disease with this powerful new prevention program

ANTIOXIDANT REVOLUTION

KENNETH H. COOPER, M.D.
AUTHOR OF *Controlling Cholesterol* AND *Aerobics*

A REVOLUTION IN PREVENTIVE MEDICINE—DR. KENNETH COOPER'S *Antioxident Revolution*!

Dr. Kenneth H. Cooper has been the groundbreaker in preventive medicine for the past three decades. He is the father of the worldwide aerobics movement, and he showed millions how to control cholesterol and hypertension. Now he takes the latest scientific antioxidant research from around the world and his own famed Cooper Clinic to bring you a simple, four-step life plan that will change your life for the better. It's revolutionary . . . and it's the simplest plan yet to build your own personal defense system that offers a longer and healthier life! You can

- reduce the risk of cancer, cataracts, and heart disease.
- delay the onset of premature aging.
- power up your immune system to fight disease.

Thomas Nelson Publishers, 1994
ISBN 0-7852-7525-8

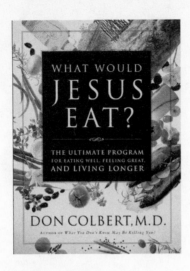

THE CHRISTIAN MARKET IS FLOODED WITH DIET AND EXERCISE programs, each claiming to be "God's way" to healthy living. While some of them are based on biblical principles, and some have even proven effective for weight loss, there is not one program leading the pack daring to answer the question *What Would Jesus Do?* Or better yet, *What Would Jesus Eat?*

This comprehensive eating plan examines Scripture and reveals what we *know* Jesus ate and what we can confidently infer He ate. Using current medical research, *What Would Jesus Eat?* demonstrates why the diet Jesus followed is ideal for twenty-first century living as well. Readers will

- understand why foods forbidden in the Old Testament dietary laws are unhealthy for us.
- learn how to follow Jesus' eating model with foods that are available today.
- realize the health benefits of the food Jesus ate and the health risks of the food He avoided.

The second half of the book equips the reader with tools to effectively follow the plan — recipes, nutritional information, and practical advice.

For those desiring to safely lose weight and for those seeking a healthier, Bible-based eating program, the only question to ask is, *What Would Jesus Eat?*

Thomas Nelson Publishers, 2002
ISBN 0-7852-6567-8